TWO-WEEK WAIT:
Motherhood
Lost and Found

Dr. Christina Greer
Rhetorica Media

Copyright © 2015 by Dr. Christina Greer.

All rights reserved. This book or any portion thereof may not be reproduced or used in any manner whatsoever without the express written permission of the publisher except for the use of brief quotations in a book review.

First Printing, 2015

ISBN-10:098615010X

ISBN-13:978-0-9861501-0-4

Rhetorica media

142 Edgington Lane

Wheeling, WV 26003

For my cub, Tristan.
You were worth the wait.

Contents

March 2010 1
April 2010 40
May 2010 53
June 2010 75
July 2010 101
August 2010 134
September 2010 173
October 2010 196
November 2010 211
December 2010 225
January 2011 242
February 2011 255
March 2011 268
April 2011 275
May 2011 284
About the author xi

Acknowledgments

THANK YOU TO EVERYONE who supported me in my journey to have a healthy child.

To my good friend and fellow writer, Kim Adams Francis, for putting up with my late night questions and for giving me the best advice in the world, even if I chose to ignore it sometimes.

To my editor, Gail Seymour, who treated my story like she would her own. Your feedback and keen eye has been indispensable

To all of the wonderful followers of my blog, Infertile Myrtle. There would be no book without you. Knowing that you were reading along on every step of my journey made me keep on writing, even when it was painful. I will be forever grateful for you kindness and support

To my students, Samantha, Keeley, Amanda, Nora, Clara, Erika, (and Arjay, too!), Priscilla, and Steve. Thank you for caring about me, my journey, and the Cub.

To my husband and co-parent, Jim. In more ways than one, I could not have done this without you. You are a great father to our son.

And to my beloved children, Samantha and Nicholas. I will miss you as long as I draw breath.

Preface

It's 5:30 am on a Tuesday morning. I am writing while my son is sleeping next to me. We are in his room on the glider, where he fell back to sleep with his head on my lap after an early morning nightmare. His face is relaxed now, peaceful. The monsters have gone. I pause every paragraph or two to watch the easy rise and fall of his chest under his Spiderman pajama top and repeat my gratitude list, which has become like a mantra for me: "He is here. He is mine. Thank you."

Five years ago when I began blogging about my journey to motherhood at [In]fertile Myrtle, my son was just a theory, a hope on a vision board. At that point I had been trying to bring a healthy child home for nearly two decades. I started blogging because it is what I do. Writing is what I have always done to survive life's struggles. I had no idea then that other people would become so incredibly invested in my story.

My original followers were friends who loved my writing and supported my efforts, but soon a quiet readership of strangers began to grow. Each entry seemed to gather more comments and likes, and I found myself drawing on that energy as I made my way through what would become my final year of trying to conceive. Although I may have written the Two-Week Wait at some point in my writing career, it would have lacked the immediacy that blogging demands. If you hadn't been reading, dear friends, this book would not exist in this form. Your responses and silent presences made this book an exciting page-turner. For that, I will always be grateful. Knowing that someone cared enough to log on each day and read my words was humbling and inspiring. I hope this book reflects that beautiful, symbiotic relationship.

If you are new to my journey, don't worry, you will get caught up in no time. I have added many reflective entries that explore the origins of my motherhood quest and the many years that followed.

If you are trying to conceive, know that I am sending you all of my best as you struggle through the agonizing days of the two-week wait. I wish you luck. Remember that a grateful heart is a full heart.

As the dawn light creeps in around the window shades, my son's face becomes more solid, material. Giving birth to him did not erase 20 years of child loss and heartbreak, but it did start the healing process. Infertility is traumatic, and the longer the struggle, the more painful it becomes. I will not tell you "I have PCOS and I did it, and so can you!" I will not say, "Keep going! It is worth the wait!" Only you know how much you can endure. I will say, however, that being a mother is more wonderful than I ever dreamed. Even nearly four years after I first saw him in the flesh, his tiny voice calling me "Mama" reminds me of how fortunate I am.

Enjoy the book. The highs and lows and everything in between. I wrote this book so I would not feel alone, and I hope by reading it, you will feel the same.

March 2010

My Struggles with Infertility

March 9, 2010 at 3:08 pm

I HAVE BEEN DEBATING on starting a blog about my struggles with infertility for some time. It is not something that I keep to myself, but being forced to write about the daily highs and lows that go along with this all-consuming challenge seemed daunting. However, I have come to a point in my quest where writing about it might be my only refuge. Although I remain hopeful, there are many dark days along this road. I am hoping this blog will give me the forum that I have always depended on for clarity and relief...writing. Here I will detail my doctor's appointments, conception strategies, and feelings as I continue waiting for a child.

My journey thus far is a long one. It begins with the birth of my first child, Samantha, in 1991. I was 17 years old. The pregnancy was perfect. She was perfect, weighing in at 8 lbs, 12 oz.

Unfortunately, she was murdered by her father when she was three and a half months old. I plan to blog about this time period on a slow day, but for the moment, I want to include this tragic time in my life because I began my quest to have another child then. But from that point on, conceiving and carrying a child to term was incredibly difficult.

After remarrying, my second husband and I conceived our son, Nicholas, who was born at 24 weeks gestation. He had implanted too low in my uterus, and by the fifth month, we knew that it was a full placenta previa, which means that the placenta was completely covering my cervix. As is common with complete previas, as my uterus grew with Nicholas, the placenta tore away from the wall of my uterus, and eventually, blood clots formed under the placenta. On March 5, 2001, Nicholas was born through emergency C-section after I nearly bled to death from a placental abruption. He lived for only one week. His complications were severe. (More on my sweet boy later.)

Following Nicholas' birth, I got pregnant two more times. The first time was an ectopic pregnancy (conceived with clomid) and the second time was a blighted ovum (conceived through low carb dieting). It has been three and a half years since I was pregnant last.

Not long after a house fire, which killed my six cats, my second husband and I divorced. I began dating my college boyfriend, and we were married just this past August. We began trying to conceive in September 2009.

Today, I am on my sixth round of Femara. I just ovulated two days ago, so the jury is still out on this cycle, which is my 53rd recorded cycle. I have Polycystic Ovarian Syndrome, which makes it even harder at 36 years of age to get pregnant.

Welcome to my blog. I hope that inscribing this journey in a public forum will help others and me as I stumble along on this path to bringing a healthy child home.

Rocks in My Pocket

March 10, 2010 at 1:15 am

ALTHOUGH I OVULATE on my own, my reproductive endocrinologist at UPMC suggested I take Femara, an anti-estrogen drug used to prevent the return of breast cancer in survivors. A side effect of the drug is that it produces ovulation and keeps progesterone levels up, which is important for women suffering with PCOS. We have chronically low progesterone. (It also causes severe depression, which I had the last time I was on it, too. Most of that I have managed to control with supplements this time around.)

I am on my sixth cycle of Femara with good results (I have ovulated each time), but still no conception. Two of those cycles I ovulated on my left side, which is the side with the fully blocked fallopian tube, and one of the cycles, dh wasn't around during ovulation. He's a truck driver and on the road much of the week. In other words, two out of six cycles so far have been viable. The word is still out on this cycle. I am two days past ovulation today, according to my ovulation predictor kit.

I was hoping to conceive on the third or fourth round of Femara, like I did on Clomid in the past, but I guess my age is really an important part of this process. Depending on who's stats you read, my chances of conceiving each month is around 10%, and even less so with the blocked tube. According to my favorite site, FertilityFriend.com,

The cumulative conception rate for women aged 35-39 is 60% after one year of trying and 85% at two years (Taylor 2003). While this may not sound so promising when you want to have a baby right now, these figures may be higher for women who are able to identify their fertile time and focus intercourse within the fertile window.

In other words, it may not be that dire, but I can tell you, after 53 cycles with no baby, it seems pretty serious!

After having the fourth cycle of Femara, I began to once again focus on alternative means of getting pregnant. I have lost 100 pounds, but I need to lose about 80 more to be at what I know is a good weight for me. It is incredibly difficult for women with PCOS to lose weight and even harder for us to keep it off, so this journey has been a long and psychologically difficult one. So, I re-focused my energy on tightening up my South Beach eating plan (that is how I lost 100 lbs in four years) and dh bought me a Wii Fit for Christmas. About three weeks ago I started working with a personal trainer, too. Most of all, I absolutely love swimming laps, and try to do it daily.

Meanwhile, I started reading about Reiki and its benefits for women with infertility. I read this great article from the UK about Reiki and conception. In it, the author claims that it is beneficial because it relaxes the body. Stress has an incredibly negative effect on conception and pregnancy, so I thought I would give it a shot. I found a local Reiki healer (more on how I found her later), and she worked on me for two hours, first with reflexology and then with Reiki. In short, Reiki is a type of hands-off healing that focuses the energy of the healer onto the receivers body. I felt great afterwards. Since then, she has also done hot stone massage. I plan on seeing her again for guided meditation...maybe later this week.

I am also interested in talismans and other totems that might help me on my journey. (Hey, why not?), so yesterday I walked down to the little gems and rock shop on my street. (Can you believe I have a gems and rocks shop on my street!?!?!) and bought two stones that are said to help with infertility: unakite and chrysoprase. The idea is that I am supposed to carry the rocks in my pocket. (Pics of these stunning pieces later.) For years, I carried a worry stone, so this didn't seem too far fetched to me. I also bought a salt votive. It is made out of halite and when illuminated is supposed to pull impurities from the air.

On the way back from my walk tonight, I stopped to swing on the swings at the playground across the street from the aforementioned gems and rocks shop. It was joyful, like always. Usually, being around children makes me a little sad, though. They are often reminders of my lack. But I heard a Mom call her boy's name, and I knew immediately that if I am pregnant with or become pregnant with a boy I want to name him Zander. It is a nice, strong name. But I am sure dh will want to weigh in on that.

Wish in One Hand . . .

March 10, 2010 at 4:01 pm

I HAVE BEEN READING about the power of wishing, which in many ways requires giving up a belief in control and being willing to accept that the universe might yield something different than what I wished for. I learned that wishes are more powerful if the wisher makes them concrete–speaks them aloud, writes them on a mirror, makes a wish box.

I began by simply Googling wishing and learned about wishing strategies and found websites where a person could submit his or her wish. I stumbled upon wishing spells, wishing talismans and stones, and wish boxes. I decided to make a wish box because it appealed to the crafter side of me (and I had a week off from work because of bad weather). Remember those dioramas in a shoe box that we made back in grade school? That's kind of what a wish box looks like, but it is about what you wish to happen and not about the story of Thomas Edison. (I drew the topic from a hat!)

I began working on my wish box by thinking about images that I wanted to include. I am wishing for a healthy child, so it seemed that I should include images of babies in my box. I began collecting pictures of babies (mostly drawings), but something just didn't seem right. Even though most of the books and articles I read about wishing insisted that wishes needed to be as specific as possible, it just didn't seem reasonable. (In my case, down to the baby's hair color, eye color, etc.) This seemed like asking the universe for far too much. I just want a healthy baby!

So I turned my focus to images of baby lions. Although that might seem strange, it made sense to me once my thoughts went down that path because I have referred to dh as my lion for ages. When we met, he had a mane of fiery red hair and he still ROARS his way through life. (For good and ill.) Off I went to the craft store (a weakness of mine) to purchase the necessary supplies. I struggled with the box (size and shape), background, 3-D elements, and even the lion cub. I selected and rejected so many items during that three hours that I think the employees thought I was going to steal something. Meanwhile, the snow started piling up.

Finally, I got home and started on my box late, late that night. I assembled my materials (all $70 worth) and made the background and a tree (out of modeling clay), but none of the lion cubs I bought seemed right. Some of them were too clownish. Others were too big or too small. I went to google images and found my favorite lion cub of all time (I have been admiring him for a year or more) and decided to use him (and the lion cub in my heart) for inspiration. As I began to draw, I was shocked at what appeared. I am NOT an artist. Previously, the height of my drawing abilities were stick people...with top hats. As this little cub appeared under my hand, I was so excited that I couldn't stopped giggling. I put my tree together, glued it all down, then went to bed.

My wish box now sits on my dresser, so that I can see this little cub's face every morning when I wake up and every night before I go to bed. Dh thinks that the wish box is "primitive art," while I think it is a laying bare of my heart's desire. I am sharing it here:

In her book, The Wishing Year, Noelle Oxenhandler goes on a wishing journey. She wishes for a home of her own, a better spiritual life, and a man with whom to share her life. By the end, she gets them all and along the way, she learns quite a bit about wishing from many different cultures. Although I found her book a bit dry (much of it could have been cut), I enjoyed the wishing quest and learned much about wishing, including the joy in wishing for others' wishes.

More on Oxenhandler's book (and some others) in my next post. For now, I wish that Grace feels better.

The Dreaded 2ww

March 10, 2010 at 11:01 pm

I AM NOW THREE DAYS past ovulation (3 dpo) and am fully engulfed in the dreaded two week wait (2ww). It is the time after ovulation and before menstruation (Aunt Flow [AF] or Time of the Month [TOM]). For women who are trying to conceive (ttc), it is absolutely terrible. (And I suppose women who are trying not to get pregnant [pg] have a good bit of trouble then, too.)

The 2ww is so awful for those of us who are in touch with our bodies and our cycles because every little body signal makes us wonder if we are pregnant. I have memorized all of the early pregnancy signs and since I have been pregnant four times, I try to remember back to those times, and all I remember is being very, very ill and having extremely tender breasts with all four. TTC women go crazy during the 2ww, and we start to wonder if our bodies are trying to betray us by sending us false signals. In reality, the symptoms women feel in early pregnancy are very similar to the symptoms women feel in the days leading up to our periods.

HOWEVER, even knowing all of that does not prevent women from obsessing over their symptoms during the 2ww. For example, last cycle I had NO symptoms at all during the 2ww, and I took that for a sign that I was pregnant for sure. After all, what I experienced was completely different than any other cycle. Alas, I just wasn't pregnant.

Right this very minute, my breasts are tender, which I KNOW is a sign of impending menstruation, but I also know that it is one of the top signs for me (and most women) of early pregnancy. Still, I can't stop thinking about it because I can't stop feeling it!

The increasing sensitivities of home pregnancy tests (hpts) compound this angst. According to my favorite site in the universe,

PeeOnaStick.com, the tests can detect levels of hcg (the "pregnancy hormone") at lower levels than ever before, which encourages (DRIVES) women like me to test so very early in the 2ww. I think I suffer this situation even more than others because of my previous ectopic pregnancy and other complications. The faster I find out I have a viable pregnancy, the safer it is for me and baby. Nonetheless, even the most sensitive of these tests are not useful for the majority of women until 12 dpo at the earliest! But there I go...peeing on the stick as early as 8 dpo based on "symptoms."

I am hoping, though, as I work through this blog this 2ww that I would be able to stave off my incredible urge to pee on a stick. It only makes things worse—seeing that single line on the stick where I hope there will be two! I really need to give myself a break. Usually, I can hold off until AF comes, but this is cycle #53, and it gets harder and harder to fight off the desire.

Wishing, Part Deux

March 11, 2010 at 12:40 am

As I mentioned earlier, I have been reading a great deal about wishing. I just finished Noelle Oxenhandler's memoir, The Wishing Year. Perhaps the most interesting parts of this book had to do with wishing strategies. I wanted something I could try out, kind of like my wish box.

One of the first tools she tried was writing what she wished for on a slip of paper and putting it between her mattress and box springs. She was very specific about what she wanted in a life partner, and she wrote down the details carefully. I have not tried this approach, and I am not sure why. I am guessing it has to do with fear of being greedy and of failure. (More on this below.) It would be simple enough to do. I guess tonight I will give it a shot. Here is what I will write: I wish to have a healthy child. He or she will be Jim's biological child and of me born. I will survive the birth and live to raise him or her and get to know my future grandchildren.

I used to think that asking for so much is greedy, but Jack Canfield and Mark Victor Hansen (authors of Chicken Soup for the Soul, which I haven't read, and The Aladdin Factor, which I have) convinced me that believing that wishing for what you want is greedy is a function of culture. Many of us are taught that asking for what you want and need is a sign of weakness and entitlement.

Oxenhandler muses on the specificity of wishing by focusing on the possibility of failure. She says,

When we wish, we aspire–and thus we can fall. Even though my paper wish is buried underneath my bed, it's my way of aiming high: for that handsome, witty, spiritually oriented, and very intelligent man. And if he doesn't come–soon–there's something about having so explicitly articulated my longing that is going to make me feel both more alone and more foolish than I did when I started.

I understand Oxenhandler's reluctance here. I have had my hopes up many times before only to be disappointed when what I wished for did not come to fruition. (Be prepared for an upcoming post on the dreaded two week wait.) However, given that everything else I have tried has failed, I am willing to take the risk.

Later, she quotes from Paul Pearsall's book, Wishing Well: Making Your Every Wish Come True. He has established a formula for wishing that goes like this:

1. SD-SU-CD–Sit Down, Shut Up, and Calm Down.
2. Pick a wish target, which means to connect and resonate with nature by looking at something alive.
3. Close your eyes.
4. Breathe deeply and abdominally.
5. Place your left hand over your heart.
6. Press your right hand gently but firmly on your left hand.

7. On exhaling, whisper your wish.
8. Use eight short words.

Oh yes, I followed those steps and whispered my wish. Now the waiting . . .

I have never been good at waiting, but I am learning how to at least not be overwhelmed by it. In fact, I have learned that good things happen while you wait, which is a pun on the old saying, but it is true. Many times in my life I have waited for something to come about and not lived my life fully in the interim. These days I try to live fully in each day for there are many little joys in it. Yesterday, I went for a swing on the swings at the park down the street. Today, I had lunch with a good friend and went for a long walk in the (these days) rare sunshine afterwards. Daily life is far too good to be spoiled by the darkness of waiting angst.

Grieving My Son

March 12, 2010 at 3:59 pm

THIS ENTRY WAS SUPPOSED to be posted yesterday, but technical difficulties interceded.

Nine years ago today my son Nicholas died. He was one week old. This entry is devoted to him and to all of the mothers out there who have suffered through child loss.

My ex-husband, Nick, and I planned on starting a family not long after we got married in 1999, but given that I had learned just the year before that I have Polycystic Ovarian Syndrome (PCOS), we expected the journey to be a long one. I tried Clomid, but it only made me anxious. (More on that in a later entry.) Then, in the fall of 2000, I felt sick for weeks. It was as though I had a lingering flu that went on for weeks. I was barely able to drag myself to work and school. On September 26, I took a pregnancy test, not really expecting to see those coveted pink lines, but there they were. I was pregnant.

Nick and I were thrilled, and we began planning on our child's birth, including shopping for baby clothes and toys. Then the bleeding began . . .

One afternoon I was sitting on the couch and felt a hot liquid pour out of my vagina. I looked down to see a thick, red fountain of blood on my pants, on the couch, on the carpet. I rushed to the doctor and discovered that I had something called placenta previa. Placenta previa is a condition in which the placenta covers the cervix. My previa was complete, meaning that it covered my cervix entirely. Placenta previa is a dangerous condition for mom and baby, but I didn't understand that then. My doctor seemed hopeful, sending me away with calming words that "at least a clot didn't form under the placenta" and that "some previas resolve themselves as the baby and placenta grow."

That is not what happened.

On March 5, 2001 at around 3 am I got out of bed because I couldn't sleep. (His gestational age was only 24 weeks.) I decided to make a baked potato and read a book. Shortly after I put the potato in the microwave, I began bleeding...five times as much as the last time. I ran to the bathroom and screamed for Nick to help me. By this time, there was a wide trail of blood from the living room through the kitchen and into the bathroom. The toilet, my socks, and the bathroom rug were coated with blood. I knew that I was in trouble. More frightening, I knew that Nicholas was, too.

Nick and I sped to the hospital. The bleeding continued. I had put a bath towel between my legs, but I bled right through it. By the time I got to the hospital, I was weak and scared. The put me in a bed and called my doctor, who at first did not believe that I was bleeding as much as I had claimed. I overheard a nurse confirm, "Yes, doctor. You must come immediately." By the time my doctor's partner arrived, I could hear the nurse's shoes sticking to my blood that coated the floor around the bed.

When he stuck the speculum into my vagina to get a better look, an enormous fountain of blood gushed out onto the bed. Nick squeezed my hand tighter, and I have never been more thankful that I could not see what was happening. They were monitoring Nicholas, but feared the worst. Minutes later, they were pushing me into surgery. I remember very clearly thinking as they pulled my bed through the double doors: "God, if this is my time to go, that's okay. I am a peace with it." Meanwhile, my anxious thoughts were focused on my son.

I woke up from the emergency C-section to find a priest I knew well and my doctor at the foot of my bed. I assumed I was dying. I asked for my son, but he was in an incubator down the hall with his father by his side. They were prepping him for flight to the nearest Children's Hospital, which was two hours away by car. I was in and out of consciousness, but eventually, they wheeled me down the hall to where they were readying his incubator for the heli-pad. I got to see my son for the first time at that moment, and I shut down. I knew then and maybe even before that that my son would not survive.

They kept him under a sheet of Saran wrap to keep him warm.

Later that night, after Nick drove to the hospital to be with our son, I cried and cried and cried. A nurse checked on me, but there was nothing anyone could do. I have never felt more helpless than that. I tried to leave the hospital immediately, but could not stand on my own. The blood loss had weakened me. They tried to force me to take a blood transfusion. I refused. A transfusion would have meant a mandatory hospital stay. I had to go to be with my son.

That evening, two nurses took me into the bathroom to clean up the long, broken rivulets of blood that still streaked my legs, and just as I was about to pass out from the pain of the C-section and the weakness from the bloodless, I saw a bright light in the distance. In the light, I saw a little girl with long hair walking hand-in-hand with a little boy with bowed legs. (Nick has bowed legs.) I knew that Samantha had come to take her brother home. Although Nicholas was alive at that moment, I took great comfort in knowing that when his time came to go that she would be there to take care of him.

He was only as long as his Daddy's hand, but he seemed bigger than the world to me.

The three of us spent an agonizing week in the NICU. His condition changed from hour to hour. One night they called us to his side because he had turned black and was surely to die, but he somehow made a rebound. He fought on and on. He was on the highest dose of pain medication possible, and yet he was still conscious a good deal of the time. I remember how his little eyes would focus on the sound of my voice as I moved from one side of his incubator to the next.

He was small, just 1 lb. and 1 oz. at birth, but he seemed so big to me.

I tried to not see the tubes and wires that kept my boy alive. I tried to just see my beautiful son.

There were so many hard parts about that week. Watching as they stuck enormous needles into his tiny abdomen to extract excess fluid. Feeling frustrated that other women—nurses—were doing things for him that I should be doing: changing his diaper, washing his face. And pumping my breast milk to be put into storage for that one day when he might be able to eat. Perhaps worst of all, I never got to hear him cry. Nick said he wailed as he came out of my womb, but I was unconscious at the time. I would do anything to hear the sound of my son's voice, just for a moment.

By the end of the week, it had become clear that he was going to die. He had had daily blood transfusions, multiple surgeries to repair the whole in his digestive tract, his circulatory system was still open, and he was on the last available means of respiratory support. One of the surgeons came to his bedside to perform emergency abdominal tapping. I asked him flat out, "Is my son going to die?" He looked me straight in the eye, and said, "Yes." Nick and I talked with the nurses and after many long hours of struggle, we knew what we had to do.

At 1:15 pm on March 11, 2001, the nurses unhooked him from the many machines and tubes that were keeping him alive and placed my son in my arms. It was the first and last time I got to hold him, but we were certainly not strangers. He was warm from the incubator, and as I looked into his beautiful eyes I told him, "I am sorry, Nicholas, but we have to let you go." Moments later, my dearest son, "Our Little Bunny," died.

When the nurse took him from me to hand him to Nick, I screamed a scream of eternal pain that I am sure was an echo of all mothers who had lost their children. We were all one in that moment of deep anguish. His warm spot stayed with me for the rest of the day and eventually gave way to an open, gnawing pit of grief that incapacitated me for months and months to come.

Despite this incredible grief, I knew then as I know now how lucky I was to have had that week with my son. Some women don't even get that. And to spend a week looking into his sweet face and memorizing every inch of his tiny person was a gift like no other. He knew his mom and his dad, and I know that he knew just how very much he was loved.

I measure his milestones as I do his sister's. I think of all of the wonderful things he could have brought to this world, knowing that he gave me the greatest gift of all: a chance to be with him and to love him, if only for the shortest of whiles.

I miss you every single day of my life, Nicholas. Now stop teasing your big sister! (I'm still his Mom, you know.)

God, Goddesses, and Other Helpmates

March 14, 2010 at 12:56 am

I JUST STARTED READING *The Healing Power of Prayer* by Chester Tolson and Harold Koenig. I am not very far into it yet, but from what I understand, the authors believe that connecting with God can help mend the mind/body split, which can lead to healing everything from physical ailments to disorders of the mind. Mostly, they argue about the relationship between stress and illness, noting that

Many specialists in the field now agree that menstrual disorders and male impotence may be the result of stress-related problems.

Although they would get Fs in one of my writing classes for not properly citing their sources, many people I have seen for infertility have mentioned the relationship between stress and the ability to conceive and maintain a pregnancy. Therefore, these fellas might be on to something. In fact, my reason for seeking Reiki therapy, herbs, and massage was to relieve some of the stress in my life. Ironically, most of the stress comes from trying (and failing) to get pregnant.

I was raised in a household that believed in God, but I never quite knew what that meant. Therefore, prayer was not a part of my coping strategies as a child. We did not attend church, and I learned about God and Christianity by tagging along with my friends' families. I was curious about The Bible (we had a couple of unread copies in the house) and by the foreign world of Church. During certain times in my life (the murder of my daughter, for one), I found great comfort in other people's faith in God. I am still more likely to ask other people to pray for me than to pray for myself. I guess I get stuck in what I call the prayer cycle. That is, if I pray for something to be different (that a loved one overcome their illness, that a friend learns to cope with her broken marriage) that it might not matter if that is not what God wants. I walk away from prayer feeling frustrated and more helpless than before I started.

At the same time, I really do believe that prayers help, but often in a way least expected. For example, when Nicholas was in NICU, people across the globe were praying for him and for our little family. I found great comfort in knowing that prayers were being sent into the universe from dozens of different religious paths. I imagined all of that good energy surrounding us as we struggled on our journey. Although Nicholas died, I do believe that I was able to not completely fall apart because of the strong embrace of those prayers. I guess I have come to believe that a higher power does exist. It may not be the Christian God or the many gods of Hinduism or Wicca's natural life force, but I think there must be something bigger than me, than you, than all of us.

Given this belief, which doesn't seem exclusive to me, I have come to see that perhaps it is possible to draw from different spiritual paths to seek strength. Maybe some people might think that this is blasphemy, heresy, or just idiocy, but I have come to realize that getting to know multiple spiritual paths helps me better understand the beliefs of others. I suppose, though, I could be accused of posing, dilettantism, or even mocking people of faith, but I am really just looking for peace and a way to live more mindfully.

A few months ago, I wandered into a local herb and incense shop with two of my good friends. I asked the owner, a Wiccan priestess, for help with herbs and oils that might help me conceive. She recommended lavender and rose oils for relaxation and red raspberry tea for strengthening my uterus. As I gathered my supplies, I wandered around the store, admiring the large selection of herbs, incense, and books. And then I saw her—the Venus of Willendorf.

I had read a bit about her years ago, but I had forgotten all about her until I found her there on a top shelf above some books on animal spirits. I was immediately captivated by her. After all, I look like her! Really, our body types are quite similar. I couldn't

God, Goddesses, and Other Helpmates

help but think that maybe this Earth mother might be able to help me on my ttc journey. I left the store with that terra cotta beauty and found a place for her on my nightstand.

Not much is known about the Venus of Willendorf. She was originally discovered in 1908 near the town of Willendorf, Austria. According to Professor Christopher L. C. E. Witcombe of Sweet Briar College in Virginia, she dates back to 24,000 to 22,000 BCE. On his great website, Women in Pre-history, he describes this early example of a human figure:

> The beginning of "history" – the shift from the prehistoric to the historic, a step marked by the advent of writing – also marks for some the move from the primitive to the civilized. The Willendorf figurine nicely illustrates the contrast. Her bulging, bulbous body, large breasts, ample abdomen, and vulva slit manifest unrefined, uncivilized, "primitive" taste.
>
> She also exhibits, in ways that are at once appealing (to most women, perhaps) and threatening (to most men, perhaps), a physical and sexual self that seems unrestrained, unfettered by cultural taboos and social conventions. She is an image of "natural" femaleness, of uninhibited female power, which "civilization," in the figure of the Classical Venus, later sought to curtail and bring under control.

Later, he goes on to say that the original naming of her as a Venus was a nasty male joke. She was not thin and modest like the desired woman of the time, but quite the opposite. Referring to her as a Venus was simply a way for men in power at the time to mock open and wild female sexuality.

But the joke certainly seems to be on them. Women and men have embraced the Venus of Willendorf as a powerful symbol of femininity, fertility, motherhood, and strength. Further, Witcombe adds:

A more common explanation is that because the statuette served as a fertility idol, the sculptor included only those parts of the female body needed for the conception and nurture of children. Even if she had feet, though, it seems unlikely that she was meant to stand up. This is even more true of the other Paleolithic figurines.

He concludes that "On the basis of this assumption, it has been suggested that, unlike today, women played a considerably more important, if not dominant, role in Paleolithic society; that possibly a matriarchy existed and women ruled."

Although I plan to continue reading about my look-alike Venus, I have also found other helpmates in my ttc journey. I have found that once I made my wish known that answers came to me in the form of suggestions for doctors to see, medications to take, and exercises to be practiced. Most significantly, I have discovered that if I let go and open myself up to the universe, help arrives.

I've never wanted to learn how to fly an airplane or to jump out of one, but I believe in the power of spiritual flight. Like Milkman in Toni Morrison's Song of Solomon, I am searching for a means to fly, to really be free because worry and fear controls my life. His best friend (and later enemy), Guitar, says, "Wanna fly, gotta give up all the shit that weighs you down." I am trying hard to do that. For me, it doesn't mean giving up material things (never been into acquiring stuff), but like Milkman, learning to fly is about purging myself of the burden of believing that I can control anything in my life. This does not mean that I should or will sit back and do nothing, but I need to learn that few things are in my control.

I believe I can fly.

Ovarian Cysts and Other Calamities

March 14, 2010 at 3:51 pm

ON WEDNESDAY, MARCH 3, 2010 (CD 12), I suffered the worst ovarian cyst pain I have ever experienced. I barely made the one-hour drive home from work. Usually, the pain from such a ruptured cyst eases by morning, but this one did not. The pain finally eased by late evening on CD 13, only to crank up again during ovulation (CD 15 and 16). I thought the cyst was healed or completely gone until Thursday, when the pain returned. The pain is much, much less severe at this point, but I haven't gone to see the doctor yet.

Ovarian cysts are common in women of reproductive years, and there are many different types of ovarian cysts.

Fortunately, through diet and exercise, I have managed to clear my ovaries of these cysts and my ovaries appear normal on ultrasound. However, since ovulation is incredibly painful for me each month (referred to as *mittleschmerz*), obviously the hard shell on my ovary that accompanies PCOS remains.

Now, I am beginning to wonder if this particular cyst is the result of six months of Femara treatment or just a fluke. In any case, I have decided to call my doctor for a Tuesday morning appointment if the pain isn't completely gone by tomorrow afternoon. I need to go in for some blood work to confirm ovulation anyway, so this will be a good opportunity to do so.

I am worried more than usual with this cyst pain because of how long it has lasted. I am hopeful that it is a corpus luteum cyst and that there is a fertilized egg implanted in my uterus, but I think it would be too early for that (just seven days past ovulation). In any case, I plan to monitor it. In addition to the one-sided pain, I now have nausea and back pain. I am not so much concerned about the impact of the cyst on my immediate health but on my future fertility. Some cysts can grow very large and can cause the ovary to contort, and this is on my good side! (The side with the open tube.)

Stay tuned . . .

A Visit to My Endo

March 15, 2010 at 6:33 pm

THE OVARIAN CYST PAIN has persisted, so I broke down and made an appointment to see my endocrinologist tomorrow morning. I have to leave here at 6 am to make it to her office by 8. First, they will do a transvaginal ultrasound, then I will chat with my doctor. If all looks okay, I will talk to her about IVF.

The IVF conversations will not be an easy one to have. I have been avoiding it for awhile because I never really considered it a possibility because of a lack of funds, but now that it is a real possibility, I am going to inquire more about it. I need to know information, like success rates and shared risk programs and all of that. I am nervous about it, and really wish that my husband would go to this appointment with me. It is not a conversation I want to have alone.

I guess I have avoided the IVF conversation for other reasons, as well. Mostly because I know that it is the end of the line. If it doesn't work, then there is no chance of pregnancy. Of course, there is still adoption, but that is not the frame of mind dh is in right now. I would adopt right now if I could, but he is holding out for his own child. I understand his desire, and I would like to give him a child of his own flesh, but I would be just as happy with an adopted child.

I will update tomorrow after I get back from the appointment.

Meanwhile, I am at 8 dpo and dying to take a pregnancy test. I know that even if the egg has been fertilized, it has not implanted yet, so there is no way that I would get an accurate result. And still... my breasts are tender, I am achy and sick, I have a headache, and I am bloated. Did I mention how much I hate the 2ww?

Of Doctors and Machines

March 16, 2010 at 10:04 pm

I GOT UP AT 4:30 am this morning to get ready for what should be a one hour drive to my doctor's office, but in rush hour traffic, it takes about double that. I left early enough, though, to keep rolling, so that there was very little riding the brake and much less stress. But I was so exhausted that I had to keep my windows down to stay awake.

At 8 am, they did an ultrasound, and the tech wouldn't tell me a thing. It used to be that I was in a position on the table to see the machine and am pretty good at reading the scan at this point (this was probably ultrasound #25 or so), but my head was too low. It was incredibly painful for her to view my left ovary, like always. That swollen and blocked left tube must be in outer space and appears to have taken my ovary with it. Nonetheless, I appreciate that she tried so hard to get a clear picture of it. Most techs just give up.

After the scan, I waited another hour to see my doctor. I tried reading about IVF but found myself easily distracted by Kirstie Alley talking about her new reality show. She was on the *Today Show*, and the first word she said was "bullshit," which made me laugh. The rest of her spot was difficult to swallow because she talked about how she is once again making her struggles with weight into a money-making venture. As I sat there in the waiting room with at least five other women, many of whom were overweight as a result of PCOS, I couldn't help but wonder what they thought of this once-again vilification of fat women. I considered making small talk, but most of the women looked like I felt: warn out and a little bit sad.

Eventually, I was called into the meeting with my doctor. She said that there was no other cyst present except for the corpus luteum cyst, which is the normal byproduct of ovulation. She doesn't understand why I had so much pain this cycle, but she is certain that I ovulated, which is good. I was happy to hear this news, and then launched into my long list of questions about IVF.

Last night, I went to the bookstore and bought In Vitro Fertilization: The A.R.T. of Making Babies by Sher, Davis, and Stoess. I knew that if everything looked good on the ultrasound that I would want to talk to my doctor about IVF. I read just about all of it before I went to bed and the rest of it in the hospital lobby this morning. For the most part, I learned that I am a good candidate for IVF. I am under 40, ovulate on my own, etc. The unknown factor; however, is that I do not know if my uterus was damaged with the placental abruption back in 2001 or not. Plus, I do not know if the emergency C-section left scar tissue that might prevent conception.

Our next step is to do exploratory surgery in May. We had planned on doing ovarian drilling, but I went into panic about it after reading that it can cause scar tissue, which can actually prevent spontaneous ovulation and even egg harvesting later. Ovarian drilling is a procedure in which a surgeon takes a laser or a scalpel and destroys ovarian tissue. It is believed (and this still is just a belief; there are no conclusive studies) that by killing some of the ovarian tissues (and eggs, too!) that the androgen (male hormone) levels in the ovaries is reduced, which causes the woman to ovulate.

Ovarian drilling is somewhat of an old fashioned approach to treating women with PCOS, but it is still done when a woman does not respond to fertility medications. I have thought for a couple of months that I would try this option, but after reading about it, I have decided that it is not for me for the following reasons:

I ovulate already. Ovulation is not my problem.

Ovarian drilling is more effective when the woman is as close to her ideal weight as possible. (I am still pretty far from that, even with the weight loss.)

Ovarian drilling can lead to scar tissue and a build up of necrotic tissue in the ovary.

The benefits of ovarian drilling can be as long as a decade or as short as a few months.

I was drawn to this procedure since we have failed so many times with Femara and my insurance will pay for it (as a treatment for PCOS). I have reconsidered.

Instead, in May my doctor will do exploratory surgery to remove my blocked fallopian tube and to examine my uterus for damage. She will also be looking for endometriosis and other potential complications. All surgeries are risky, but this one is fairly safe. It will be laparoscopic, which means she will make an incision in my belly button and insert the tools and camera. It is like gallbladder surgery but a little further south.

After I heal from this surgery, then we begin the prep for IVF. It looks like we will do the first procedure in July or August. I am very concerned about it, but I have decided to focus my energies into reading as much about it as I can and by preparing myself for the emotional and physical toll. I will be blogging, exercising, eating healthy, relaxing, and continuing to work on strengthening my marriage.

I left there feeling hopeful (and tired). Now, we just need to come up with the money. I believe we will. We will just have to try. My husband is behind this, and I am very grateful for that. It is hard to believe that this time next year, I might be expecting our child. I plan on going to IVF orientation next month and then talking to the financing department after the exploratory surgery in May.

Meanwhile, I am at 9 days past ovulation. I have to wait a week to take a pregnancy test. If this cycle is a bust, I will do one cycle of Clomid at my request. I figure, why not mix it up?!?! It never hurts to try something else.

Hidden Meanings

March 17, 2010

YESTERDAY AFTERNOON, I visited the rock shop down the street to have the owner make me a fertility bracelet. I had seen a beautiful one online, but it was quite costly, and it seemed impersonal. I wanted to pick out the stones and the charm that would hang from it.

I chose moonstones and rose quartz, but in a different size than on the bracelet I found online. I also chose a fertility goddess charm instead of the turtle on the original bracelet. (Both are symbols of fertility.) I picked each bead and each piece of silver. My rock hound friend put it all together, and I picked up a little while ago.

It is absolutely gorgeous. I saged it, to cleanse it of negative energy, when I got home. Now I will wear it as often as I can in the hopes that the two stones will help me on my journey.

According to the all-knowing rock lady, moonstone has the following properties:

> *A stone for hoping and wishing; allowing one to recognize the 'ups and down' and gracefully acknowledge the changing cycle allowing one to sustain, maintain, and understand their destiny. Moonstone cleanses negativity and enhances the positive attributes of creative and self-expression. It is used for protection against the perils of travel and is a talisman of good fortune.*

All of those qualities should help me on my journey, especially the hoping and wishing part. And I will need the protection from the perils of travel tomorrow as I head out of state.

Once again, it sounds like a valuable stone to keep on my person. I like the idea of the stone bringing calmness. I need that right now and throughout the journey to having a child.

I guess the bracelet will give me something to hold onto, especially since the fertility goddess fits perfectly in the palm of my hand when my arm is hanging down.

Before I left the rock shop today, I asked her about the significance of Amber. Last summer, just as DH and I were picking up the pieces and trying to get our life together in order, I developed an intense love for Amber. It is a gorgeous stone, and it seems to work well with my dark hair and eyes. I wore Amber earrings and an Amber necklace on my wedding day, and a month before that I bought a gorgeous Amber ring. I had never been interested in it before then.

I could not believe that I had unconsciously been choosing Amber over and over because I needed to heal myself and because I was struggling with the choice of getting married. DH is the love of my life, and I can think of no more fitting stone to wear on our wedding day than that one.

Most interesting of all of these hidden meanings I have been uncovering is the heart I found in my yard last night. I was walking back from the rock shop, and in the corner of my yard, I saw something red. At first I passed it up, thinking it was a piece of ribbon from a child's toy, but then I went back for it. It is a simple metal heart with a red ribbon. I can't quite tell what it might have been attached to before, but I plan on attaching it to my small handbag or even my rearview mirror. It has a flower on it, which is the symbol of hope and spring and life!

I know that someone, probably a child, dropped it by accident, but I can't help but feel that I was meant to find it. I think this is a good sign.

Caving In

March 19, 2010

I AM AWAY at a conference for a few days. I have been having a great time, but my fertility situation is always on my mind.

This morning I spent some time with one of my best girlfriends. We had no specific plans and ended up going caving. My memories of caverns go back to my children, when my family would spend at least a week each summer exploring the underground of our home state. These are fond remembrances. The perfect temperature of the caverns. The darkness. The incredible rock formations. Of course, it was good to be with my family, which included my grandmother for many years. We did not get along most of the time, but being so far under the surface seemed to shut us up ... for a little while.

As we explored the vast cave system, I was stunned by the smoothness of the stones and the care that the park system has taken in managing the caves. Mammoth State Park is gorgeous, and I felt at peace there. I love hiking and spending a day in the woods, but it the humid air and quiet of the caves helped me feel more centered than I could have imagined.

At some point along the way, my friend pointed to the ceiling to show me a natural downspout from a sinkhole on the Earth's service. Water rushed out of it in a long stream for five stories to the creek below. We giggled, realizing that the formation from which the water ran was a perfectly shaped and shaded vulva. I took a picture (yet to be developed) in the hopes of connecting with this subterranean symbol of the goddess.

As we climbed farther and farther down, the womb-like feeling was unmistakable, and I found myself thinking about this journey as being a kind of descent into hell, as in the quest of the hero. Down and down I went into the darkness, uncovering with each step a quieter, more dangerous place.

We made our ascent an hour and a half later, and we stepped out into the sunlight. I felt re-born, not in a significant sense, but in that moment.

I know that there is so much more to life than this journey, but it seems to be the goal among all goals for me. I have achieved everything else I have strived for: wonderful friendships, a well-paying, meaningful career, a home, marrying my DH, and many other objectives, large and small. Becoming a mother will not make me feel whole, but I believe it will allow me to share my love, experience, and knowledge with another being.

Before leaving home on my trip south, I scheduled my surgery to remove the tube. Up until then, that surgery was theoretical, but making the appointments for pre-op, the surgery, and the post-up, drove the reality of it home. It should get me one step closer to getting pregnant, but that doesn't mean that I am not scared of the procedure and what we may learn through it.

Finding Fortune

March 21, 2010

IT SEEMS everywhere I go these days, I find something that relates to my current journey. Although I know that it is probably because I am looking, I have never experienced anything quite like this. It is as though once I opened up to the universe, the universe opened up to me.

In addition to the little heart I found in my front yard last week, I have received a fortune cookie fortune all about dreams, got to see my nephew for the first time in nearly a year, and found a giant plastic ladybug under the bar of my sun awning.

The other night my friends and I went out to dinner at a Vietnamese restaurant. After an excellent meal of green tofu in curry sauce with veggies, the time came for the reading of fortune cookies. One friend had a fortune about money, another about love, and another didn't quite make sense. Then, it was my turn to read out loud:

In order to achieve your dreams, you have to have one.

I erupted into giggles, given my recent quest with dreams and wishes. How fitting! It is as though my life philosophy was captured on that little slip of paper. Of course, this is not the first time that I have had a fortune cookie fortune relate to something pressing in my life, but given that my friends' fortunes didn't seem to fit their situations, I took mine a little bit more to heart. After all, I am in the swells of a vast dream. I have one! I do!

Then, this afternoon, my nephew and the plastic ladybug appeared.

I have been estranged from my nephews for more than a year. Their mother (my brother's ex-wife) has refused to let anyone in my family see the kids because of a grudge she carries against my brother. Today, my brother called to say that he was bringing his youngest son to visit me. At first I didn't believe him because in the past, his mother has agreed to a visit, and then changed her mind minutes before they were supposed to leave, but my mother confirmed that they were on the way.

I have grieved the loss of both boys. One of the reasons I worked so hard to move home is because I was so frustrated with having to miss football games, Valentine's parties, Christmas plays, and all of the moments in which an aunt can be so proud of her nephews. However, not long before I moved home, my brother and his now ex-wife went through a bitter breakup, and she took the kids away from all of us. They were nine and eleven at the time.

In many ways, they filled a gap that was left behind when my children died. I never saw them as replacements, but certainly as children who needed and wanted my love and support. Now, I feel their absence at each holiday, on their birthdays, and on special days in my life. It is as though I am living in a kind of limbo. They are not gone forever, but I cannot be with them. I feel like Tantalus, just inches away from what I need with no relief.

Our visit went well. He is taller and darker haired than last year, and he hugged me warmly and told me he missed me. It was hard to say goodbye to him, but I kept my smile and voice light and cheery. More than anything, I hope that he knows that he is so important to me and that despite his parents' problems, I love him and want the best for him. He'll be 12 in a few days, and he will want to spend less and less time with adults than he does now. I miss him and his brother more than I can even admit to myself.

During his visit, I unrolled the sun awning on my back deck. I looked up when it was fully open and was surprised to see two antennae poking out from behind the bar holding the awning to the house. At first I thought the bug was real, a giant moth perhaps. But as I moved closer, I realized it was a plastic ladybug. I couldn't imagine why I had never seen it before. I must have unrolled the awning a dozen times since I moved here.

My nephew climbed up on a deck chair and retrieved it from its hiding place. It has a hole in the bottom big enough to fit on a child's finger, which he promptly demonstrated. I imagine it must have fit on the top of a toy or an umbrella or the back of a child's lawn chair. It was made to be removable, so it was not broken, and it was in perfect condition.

At first I thought that perhaps a child had deliberately placed the ladybug behind the bar. As I watched my nephew, who is tall for his age, struggle to reach it, I realized the children who lived here before me could not have put it there. The oldest was a girl of about seven. I have found other mementos of their time in this house, including a picture of all three children, a Scooby Doo sticker on one of the bathroom doors, and a pair of baby nail clippers on the front porch. Clearly, this rubber insect was a long-forgotten remnant as well. I imagine that one of them tossed it up onto the awning and over repeated uses, it made its way up the awning and down to the back of the support bar.

No matter how it got there, I took it is a sign of the universe speaking to me about children, lost and found. I have had some of the first, but none of the second, until this afternoon when I found my nephew once again.

I already knew the Asian legend that if you whisper your true love's name to a ladybug, when it is released, it will fly to your love, deliver its message, and your love will come to you.

However, I was astonished to read the following at *The Doorway of Symbolism*: a ladybug can symbolize that

- A new love interest is on the way
- New love in the form of a pregnancy or new born is right around the corner
- Closer attention to loved ones is required at this time
- It's time to pursue your passion and do more of what you love
- Self-love is vital – are you loving yourself enough?

I started to dig a little further and found that other sources corroborate this meaning and go even deeper. According to *The Cycle of Power: Animal Totems:*

> *A messenger of promise, the ladybug reconnects us with the joy of living. Fear does not live within joy. The need to release our fears and return to love is one of the messages it carries.*
>
> *Ladybug teaches us how to restore our faith and trust in Great Spirit. It initiates change where it is needed the most. When ladybug appears it is asking us to get out of our own way and allow Great Spirit to enter.*

Of course, I have been trying to do just those things in my life in general, but with fertility in particular. It is hard for a person with my drive and ambition to let go, but I am getting better at it every single day.

According to the site, *Ladybug Lore,* ladybugs are considered incredibly lucky in all cultures and to kill one is considered to be bad luck. (Of course, around this part of the country, ladybug infestation is so common that many people do exterminate them.)

Of course, this site makes me want to learn more about totem animals and their meanings, but I think I will save that delightful journey for another day when I have time to explore their potential. For now, I will dwell on the often-missed clues that the universe seems to provide. Would I have saved my fortune cookie fortune this time last year? Would I have noticed the ladybug hiding beneath the support rod if I hadn't started really looking at the world around me? Would I have had the most wonderful fortune of seeing my nephew if I didn't begin to believe that the universe will provide?

I am not sure what all this means. I just know that I have been incredibly moved by each presence. It seems that as each day unfolds, I am greeted with another sign of hope that my dream, my wish, will come true. These signs give me the courage to keep dreaming, to break open a sweet treat, to believe that a mother's heart can be changed, and to look under a sun awning for hidden joys.

I gave my nephew the ladybug. He gleefully walked away with it stuck high upon his index finger. Not long ago, I would have kept it, fearing that its magic would not work if I gave it away. But I learned a lesson from that ladybug long before I looked up its meaning: Let go, Christina. It's okay.

The Arrival of Aunt Flo

March 22, 2010

IT IS THE END of one incredibly miserable day. I woke up with mild (as always) period cramps, so I knew that Aunt Flo (or TOM or whatever euphemism you wish) was on its way. I felt like crying, but I made it all the way to my car and even to the interstate before my usual morning call from my husband made me burst into tears. He said he could tell something was wrong when I answered the phone. I tried not to explain why I felt so sad, but before I knew it, I was crying and blabbering about another busted month.

He said a few kind words, but he really doesn't understand. I am the one who must live with this emotional pain month in and month out. I know he wants a child, too, but he can, in a sense, sit back and enjoy the ride. He doesn't want to attend classes with me or go to doctors' appointments. I am left to deal with my body's signals every single cycle.

It is 15 days past ovulation (DPO), I thought that it would hold off until tomorrow at least. I am usually on time all the time. Instead, by the time I taught my 1 p.m. class, my period had arrived.

When you are trying to get pregnant, the end of every cycle and the start of a new one brings on grief. I am grieving over another cycle of failure and the loss of a potential new life. It has been said that orgasms are a *la petit mort*, or little death. For me, as a woman trying to conceive (TTC), my period is such; a little death.

I know that the menstrual cycle is a sign of renewal and rebirth. It is, after all, a cycle that goes and on and on. But the arrival of menstrual blood each time simply reminds me that I am, once again, not pregnant. I am not expecting a baby. I am not going to have a child any time soon. Each cycle that is washed away by my period, reminds me of how far I am away from holding a child in my arms.

I am usually upbeat. I can see the upside of nearly everything, but I allow myself this one day each cycle to grieve. I need it. I must pause for a day and allow myself to revel in the sadness that I feel, knowing that there is no hope this cycle. It is done.

I will begin Clomid for this new cycle. It is #54. I do wonder on these grieving days how many more times I can see red and not say to myself, "STOP." After all, if I was a woman not trying to conceive, the beginning of my period would be just another day.

Jealous Thoughts

March 24, 2010

I AM SICK TODAY as I have been for the past couple of days. I have a mild fever and just general aches and pains. The right side of my face is swollen. Both of my ears are clogged. I am hoping it is simply allergies and a minor ear infection. I bought a Neti pot to clear things up, but I have yet to use it.

But today's entry is not about my ears and throat, but about my heart and the feelings of envy and jealousy that I sometimes feel when I see moms with their children.

Today, I sat at the table across from a young family. Mom, dad, and baby. I watched as the mom fed her little one strained peas, or some other jarred baby mixture. I know from experience that trying to eat your own dinner while feeding your baby his or her dinner is not pleasant. I also know from experience that there are times when it would be easier to just hide under the table for a few, quiet seconds than deal with the stress of a crying child.

At the same time, I couldn't help but feel jealous of this woman and her small child. Watching his or her tiny fingers reach out for her hand each time she took the spoon from the jar made me crave that moment. More than anything else, though, I longed to put the look on my husband's face that he had as he stole glances of the fussy baby. He was smiling. Inside, I was wailing.

I suppose jealousy is not even the right word for moments like these. Envy is perhaps better. I envied her even in that space of humdrum routine. What could be more mundane than spoon feeding an infant? But for me, it seemed like the whole world was bound up in those actions. I wished for more than a moment that I was the one with my hand covered in pureed food and baby slobber. That, my friends, is the good life.

The Children I've Carried

March 25, 2010

ON MY WAY HOME from work this evening, I heard an interview with Tim O'Brien, the author of *The Things They Carried*. O'Brien's collection of stories reflected on his time during the Vietnam War with specific meditations on the items that men carried into battle, but also on what they carried out and back across the ocean. Although I would not compare the darkness of war to trying to conceive or even to child loss, there is a similar quality to O'Brien's focus on the physical and symbolic weight of horror and tragedy.

In addition to my daughter, Samantha, and my son, Nicholas, I have been pregnant two other times. One of those pregnancies was an ectopic pregnancy and the other one was a blighted ovum. Although both pregnancies were short lived and risky to my health, I carried them and still do.

The ectopic pregnancy occurred in the fall of 2004. My ex-husband and I were trying to conceive for a few months. On our third month of Clomid, the pregnancy test came back positive. I immediately started progesterone suppositories to keep my levels up and began injecting myself with low dose heparin to prevent miscarriage.

Following the birth of my son, my doctor suspected that I had a clotting disorder. He tested me for about twenty different ones, and the only factor that came back abnormal was Factor VIII, which is responsible for breaking up blood clots.

The theory in the medical community is that if a pregnant woman with a clotting disorder administers low dose heparin (or Lovenox) to her abdomen twice a day, then it will prevent miscarriage. I was never convinced that I had a clotting disorder. The studies I read said that Factor VIII and other factors were naturally elevated after birth, so I assumed that explained it. Later, a hematologist confirmed my clotting factors were normal. But I followed my doctor's orders and ended up with a severely bruised stomach, but a potentially healthy pregnancy.

Meanwhile, as the pregnancy progressed, it became very clear that it was not a normal pregnancy. My human chorionic gonadotropin (hCG) numbers would triple and then double and then plummet, then double again. After a few weeks of testing, it became clear that the pregnancy was ectopic. Ectopic pregnancies are called so because they implant outside of the womb. Usually ectopic pregnancies implant in the tube, but they can implant anywhere in the body, including the abdomen.

We attempted to visualize the pregnancy, but like in many ectopic cases, it was never identified on ultrasound. We knew it was there only because of my wildly fluctuating numbers. Faced with no other solution, we decided that the best course of action was methotrexate, a chemotherapy agent used to kill fast growing cells.

The decision was not a hard one for me. I knew I was taking a life, but I also knew that this little life growing inside of me would kill me if it got any bigger. I knew the chance of survival for a pregnancy outside the womb was as close to zero as not being pregnant at all. I was distraught to be losing a potential life, but I also knew there really was no choice.

It was a warm October day when I went to the clinic for the methotrexate shot. The nurse showed it to me, and I recoiled from its obviously toxic, neon green glow. I went home that day, knowing the life inside me was dying to save my own. As I recovered from the transient nausea and mouth sores from the methotrexate in the days that followed, I watched as my hCG numbers fell to zero and the pregnancy was dissolved. I don't feel guilty for doing what I had to do, but I do feel tremendous loss from the life that would never/could never be. That child would be almost five years old.

A couple of months later, my house burned down, killing my six cats. The landscape of my body, my mind, and my heart had been forever changed.

We took a break after the ectopic. I was scared of it happening again. After all, a ruptured tube can be life-threatening. We began trying again in the fall of 2005. I decided to try dieting one more time before giving up for good. I chose the South Beach Diet. Within three months of going on the plan, I found out I was pregnant.

Nothing about that pregnancy was right. The embryo had implanted low in my uterus, and the diagnosis from pregnancy to natural abortion to pregnancy changed from day to day. As my doctor followed me closely on ultrasound, it became pretty clear the baby was not developing. We saw a fetal sac and what appeared to be a brain stem. At one point, we even thought we saw a heartbeat, but it was mine. Sadly, my doctor decided that it was a blighted ovum.

Blighted ovums are basically empty egg sacs. The egg and the sperm get together but do not form an embryo. According to the American Pregnancy Association,

> *A blighted ovum is the cause of about 50% of first trimester miscarriages and is usually the result of chromosomal problems. A woman's body recognizes abnormal chromosomes in a fetus and naturally does not try to continue the pregnancy because the fetus will not develop into a normal, healthy baby. This can be caused by abnormal cell division, or poor quality sperm or egg.*

In many ways, facing this loss was far harder than the ectopic because I could see something. It wasn't a baby. It was just an empty sac. But it was visible on ultrasound. And I knew then this would be the last time my ex-h and I would try. By this time, our marriage had fallen apart.

Once we realized it was a blighted ovum, my doctor sent me home to miscarriage naturally. I did pass quite a bit of fetal tissue, but it became pretty obvious my body was not going to expel it all. After about ten days of trying to miscarry on my own, I went in for a Dilatation and Curettage (D&C). That day was a dark, dark day. I cried and cried that day. I knew that there was nothing alive growing in my womb, but I felt so attached to this child-to-be. After all, I figured that it was my last hope.

I was unconscious for the D&C, and when I woke up, I found myself in a puddle of blood. I kept on bleeding heavily for many hours after I was released. When the blood finally stopped, I called my doctor and asked her about what she found in my womb during the procedure. She said, simply, "Necrotic tissue." The dead remains of a pregnancy that never really started.

In my distress, I struggled to find a way to make some kind of sense and peace with this incredible loss. I found a website for The Church of the Holy Innocents, which is located in New York City. They maintain *a Shrine to the Holy Innocents:*

> *Often children who have died before birth have no grave or headstone, and sometimes not even a name. At The Church of The Holy Innocents, we invite you to name your child(ren) and to have the opportunity to have your baby's name inscribed in our "**BOOK OF LIFE**". Here, a candle is always lit in their memory. All day long people stop to pray. On the first Monday of every month, our 12:15pm Mass is celebrated in honor of these children and for the comfort of their families.*

Knowing this gave me tremendous peace, and I filled in the certificate and gave the unborn baby that never was a baby a name: Amber Rose. I love the color amber, and she was like the loveliest of flowers, the rose. I never knew this child who would never be a child, but she was a part of me.

And these are the children I still carry.

Drastic Times Call for Drastic Measures

March 28, 2010

I AM DOWN to the wire, facing the gauntlet, biting the bullet, or whatever cliché you've got roaming around in your head. I am on my last doctor-sanctioned medicated cycle. I just started the dreaded Clomid recently, so I am in desperation mode. Basically, I will have surgery in May, and then hopefully start IVF in July. Given how terribly difficult IVF is on the body, I have decided to give an extreme measure one more chance.

Tomorrow, I begin strict low-carb dieting. It really is my last resort before IVF.

Why low carbing? I have PCOS, which is an insulin uptake disorder (among other blasted things), and I am on a moderate carb plan now, but I was able to get pregnant twice while low carbing, so I figure I can do this for 90 days.

The bad side: very, very limited food options, especially since I do not eat meat, MSG, or artificial sweeteners. Also, once I go off-plan, I will gain all the weight back and then some. No doubt about it. Plus, I will really, really miss bananas and apple. Woe is me!

Nonetheless, I know that it is probably a shot in the dark, but I have to at least try it one more time.

Wishes DO Come True

March 31, 2010

ONE OF MY FAVORITE students has a rapidly deteriorating eye condition. He is 19, and has been told by a number of specialists that he will likely be blind within the next five years. He has been given little hope of stopping the progress of the disease. At best, they can slow it.

Although there are experimental procedures available for him in China, the cost and unknown side effects have prevented him from pursing this option. He has been told by experts in the field this surgery might become available in the US within the next five years, but there is no guarantee.

Obviously, it is a tremendous challenge for a person so young to deal with the knowledge that blindness is more than likely his fate, and yet he manages to keep a positive outlook on his situation and on life in general. He is high strung and has a difficult time controlling his impulses, which might make him a challenge for some teachers, but I embrace his enthusiasm and willingness to speak his mind. He's a good kid, and I genuinely worry about his future.

Earlier this month, I had been reading about wishing. I made my wish box, put my slip of paper under my mattress, and wished and wished and wished. The material I read was illuminating in terms of helping me understand why wishing is so powerful. Common among all wishing texts is the encouragement for wishers to wish for the wellbeing of others, too. Wishing for others is good.

Soon after I finished my last wishing book, I decided to make a wish for someone else. I chose my student. I said my wish aloud and forgot all about it.

This afternoon he stopped me after class, like he always does, and told me he had good news. Three months ago, as a last resort, his doctor gave him a special kind of eye drops that he hoped would buy my student a little more vision for a little longer. It turns out his vision has improved far beyond any expectation, and even some of his other eye problems have diminished. I was so very happy to hear this news, and I immediately remembered my wish.

I said, "I wished for you!" And I told him the story about wishing and dreaming and hoping.

Whether my wish helped my student or not will never be known, but it is pretty obvious that by wishing for him, I became a bigger part of his journey. Even if wishing is not direct but associative, it still seems magical to me.

April 2010

Notes on the End of a Term

April 5, 2010

THE SEMESTER is nearly over. We have three weeks of classes left and then finals. It has been a rough term. Bad weather. Illness. Yet somehow, we are making it. Most of us, and this most definitely includes me, are just limping by, but getting by we are.

I love my students. They sometimes do not turn in their papers on time, and there are moments when I wished they would work just a little bit harder, but they are good kids. I am especially close to this year's students, partly because they were born the same year as my daughter, Samantha. This would have been her first year of college, too.

Of course, I mark the milestones in my mind: when she would have started kindergarten, when she would have gotten her driver's license, when she would have gone to prom. Although they make me a little sad when they come and go, most of the time I simply imagine how she might have been at each stage. How she might have looked or talked or acted. All supposition, of course, but I can't help but think of her on big days when I am sure I would have been so proud of her.

I have written about these moments in the epilogue to my essay, "In the Stillness of the Waiting Room," which appeared in *The*

Awakenings Review a while back. It is an essay about trying to come to terms with her murder. I was pregnant with Nicholas at the time.

> Years went by and hallucinations turned into hauntings. Her apparition has aged as she would have aged, year-by-year growing taller and braver. Her featureless form now hides in corners, emerges from doorways, and peers out from beneath beds. She appears only as a rough shape, undefined and shallow, because I can only imagine what her face would have become by this time, age ten. I cannot visualize the concrete texture of what would be the length of her hair, the slope of her shoulders, the contours of her hips.
>
> Hers is not the usual haunting. No clanging chains in the night. No cold fingers on my unsuspecting spine, but rather a quiet movement of shadow that fills up spaces that I can't quite reach. I see her walking to school, a dark outline bouncing along with the living children. I see her dancing in her first ballet recital, silently spinning in time with the piano. And I see her in the mirror some mornings, right beneath my own skin, smiling at me. Sometimes I think I hear her laughter, high-pitched and light, coming from the room that might have been hers.
>
> I am never afraid to see her. Rather, I am afraid that these apparitions will someday fade and all I will have left are these nearly-white stretch marks that line my abdomen and brief flashes of memories that may slowly be replaced with the soft, round face of my second child. As he grows larger inside me each day, I find myself trying desperately to make peace with Samantha's ghost. For the first time since her death, I am coming to terms with the loss. I have stopped lying to myself. Her death has become more real, more present. I feel a new emotion rising up to meet what remains of my grief—guilt. Guilt for

the life that I could never give her with Jason. Guilt for the better life that I know this child will have with my second husband. Guilt for somehow not knowing what was going to happen long before it did.

I feel the baby kick, his strong legs jamming tiny toes up under my rib cage. I imagine Samantha's ghost kneeling beside the chair as I read a bedtime story to her unborn brother. I hold my breath for a moment, hoping that the warm wisp of air doesn't send her spectral form into the darkness forever.

This school year the apparitions have turned into live beings. My students. When I walked in that first day of class last fall, I was struck by them. I have been teaching freshmen for 14 years now. They don't look much different now than they did back when I first began teaching. They are sweatshirts and jeans clad, baseball caps and book bags late-stage adolescents. And yet I was overwhelmed by their presences. As I got to know them, these feelings intensified.

I can't help but wonder, would Samantha wear her hair that way? Would she be smart? Would she play basketball? Would she giggle loudly at bad jokes? Would she belong to a big group of friends? Would she be a loner?

For the first time in my teaching career, I am actually old enough to be my students' mother. In some ways it is unsettling, but in many others it is incredibly enriching. I am not a parental figure to my students. I have never tried to be. I have never wanted to be. Instead, I am their mentor. I try to help them if I can, but I want them to stand on their own. I don't think of them as my children, but rather as young people who need guidance, and I try to give that to them.

There have been painful moments this year. The final project for my Honors students last term required them to make digital essays, which are short films about some aspect of their personal lives. In other words, they had to tell me a story using photos, music, and a narrated script. As I graded each story over Christmas break, I cried. Some of them were very well done. Some of them were not. All of them were beautiful. As I watched the vignettes of their lives unfold, I was struck by the vast amounts of sadness and joy that each of them had lived through in their 18 years on this Earth. I couldn't help but wonder if Samantha could make a movie about her life, would it be happy or sad?

Would my daughter have had a good life? Would she have gone off to college and told a story about her life that would have expressed the terrible sadness and incredible joy of her life? Would she love her mother? What song would my little girl sing?

As I make my way to the end of the term, which, ironically, is about nine months, I am filled with a tenderness for these kids. Like my very first class of students, I am sure I will remember them, their faces, their names, and the moments they shared with me. I wish them a happy future and hope they don't mind that when I look at them sometimes I can't help but see my daughter and what she might be today.

Clomid Craziness

April 7, 2010

FOR THE FIRST TIME since 2004, I am taking clomiphene citrate, Clomid, for ovulation. When I took it back then, it made me absolutely insane and actually set off what became a years-long battle with anxiety disorder. I took it this cycle to see if maybe, in a last ditch attempt, it might work where Femara has not. Actually, Femara has done what is should do, make me ovulate, but no conception yet.

I figured that since this is our last medicated cycle until we try IVF in July that I would try my old friend Clomid again. Well, just like last time, I am insane.

It makes my moods cycle from sadness to anger to deep, dark depression in minutes. I yell at my husband. I have an attitude at work. And I feel bloated and tired. Really. Too much fun.

The problem is that although I know what his happening when it happens, I cannot find a way to control it. Yesterday, I was absolutely out of control. I was angry at my husband because we were just about to miss my fertile window, which would make taking Clomid and acting like a jerk useless. I did not intend to be so outraged, but I was completely insane.

I believe that my emotions and behaviors would be easier to manage if he didn't drive for a living. With him out on the road, timing intercourse is nearly impossible. Some cycles he is home every night during the fertile window. Other cycles, he is not home at all! I know that he cannot help his schedule, but when he is home, I feel like he needs to do his job.

I hate to think of it that way. I love him, and making love is a very important part of who we are (and of any romantic relationship), but I get so angry when he comes home off the road and decides that he is too tired for sex. I do understand exhaustion, but I wonder if he understands what these fertility drugs are doing to my body and mind every single cycle? They are tearing me apart. I wish he didn't have to work so much. I wish he had more time to himself. I wish he could sleep more. I also think that if he has time for a two hour workout at the gym, then he should be able to have sex during the three or four day fertile window.

I look forward to IVF ONLY in that his semen sample will be frozen, and his work schedule will not interfere with ovulation timing. I do not look forward to being even more insane than I have been so far. But I still believe that all of this is for the greater good. Right?

Lions, Tigers, and Elephants?

April 18, 2010

I MADE THE MISTAKE when I was pregnant for Nicholas of buying a ton of baby clothes, toys, and other things. I couldn't have known that I was going to give birth prematurely and that he would die, but at five months of pregnancy, I should have waited to get ready for his arrival.

I am careful about that these days. However, the other day at the thrift store (I am a thrift store freak), I could not help but buy a sweet wooden elephant. It is handmade with wheels and a long green string.

The husband thought I was crazy when I showed it to him. In fact, he flat out said, "You have gone over the deep end this time." But I explained to him that although I had a future child in mind when I bought it, it is a very nice piece of primitive art. It is sitting in front of my fireplace at the moment. It looks good in our living room. I do hope someday I will hear its squeaky wheels rolling across the hardwood floors when it is being dragged along by a toddler. Of course, I have played with it, and the cats seem to enjoy it just as much as I do.

I used to collect elephants, especially wooden ones. I was drawn to their size and shape, kind of like my own, but also to the elephant's nature. It seems that they are kind creatures who mourn the loss of their loved ones, and whose memories do go back quite some time. It is hard to resist these wild beasts.

I lost my collection in the house fire in 2004, and like with most stuff I cared about then, never managed to begin collecting again. Then, I saw this wooden chap and could not resist. Besides, he was $1.99 cheap!

Of course, Ganesha, the Hindu god I mentioned in previous posts, has an elephant head, so perhaps I was drawing on his good luck and ability to bust through obstacles when I bought this red fellow.

In any case, he will sit in front of my fireplace until a kid comes along to play with him. Until then, I will be reminded of the sunny spring day when I found him and hope in a used toy bin in Pennsylvania.

Nail Biting in the 2ww

April 18, 2010

HERE I AM AGAIN, stuck in the dreaded 2ww. The good news is I only have six days left. The bad news is my symptoms are absolutely bizarre this time around. I know I probably say that all the time...

I am at 10 DPO. My fingernails, which wouldn't grow if I soaked them in Miracle Grow for a month, are suddenly long and strong. The only other time my nails have been like this is when I have been pregnant. For a while I thought that maybe the growth is due to the prenatal and other vitamins I have been taking, but surely, I would have seen this type of result before now. I have been taking them for seven months. Why this month? Why this part of the cycle?

Secondly, I cannot stop peeing. I even wake up in the middle of the night to go, which is unlike me. Of course, my breasts are tender, too, which is a confusing sign. It could be an indication of impending AF or pregnancy, so it is not reliable. Are any signs, though?

Also, I have had terrible stomach problems in the past week, which happens to me during pregnancy. And now, I have severe insomnia. It is nearly 5 am, and I am still awake!

In addition, I have had cramping off and on since 4 DPO, but I had that same issue during the first few cycles of Femara.

Finally, yesterday I woke up with the song, "New Kid in Town," by the Eagles, blaring in my head. Compelling, no?

I could take a pregnancy test this morning, but Fertility Friend says that it is only like to be 13.3% accurate if I take one so early. I will wait as long as I can, unless I see obvious signs of her arrival, such as that fluttering feeling I get right before she starts, an entire day of absolute exhaustion, that pre-period scent, or spotting.

Surely, a pee-on-a-stick addict like me can wait six more measly days, right? Right?

12 DPO and No Sign of Flo

April 20, 2010

WELL, HERE I AM in the throes of the end of the dreaded 2ww. It is almost over. Just four more days to go until this cycle craps out. Then, no more meds until IVF in July. It will be strange not to pop pills for a few months while I wait. But still, those four days will drag on and on.

As expected, I did take a couple of home pregnancy tests. Both were negative. I did not take one this morning, though. I only have two left, and I want to save them for if and when I need them.

My symptoms today: tender breasts, creamy cm, exhaustion, cramps, and still LONG fingernails. Of course, I know that it is most likely all for naught, but I am really hopeful that I got pregnant this time. I want to have a baby, and I surely don't want to have the surgery that is coming up on May 11.

Just four more days and the misery of this 2ww will be behind me.

What Would My Future Look Like If...?

April 23, 2010

WELL, AS YOU MIGHT expect from the post title, AF is on her way. Spotting two days in a row, which means the big, ole witch will be here tomorrow morning, right on time. I had such high hopes for this cycle! On the plus side, I guess this new nail growth thing is a function of my totally awesome nutrition and not pregnancy, so they are here to stay. Rock on!

Anyway, last night I had a series of mild panic attacks. I haven't had many of those since I stopped taking my meds two years ago, so it was a bit of a surprise. I think they were a result of the Clomid, but also exhaustion, stress, and AF-related hormone fluctuations.

As I lay awake, I couldn't help but focus on the fact another cycle has come and gone, and I am still not pregnant. I haven't been pregnant in four years. I might not ever be pregnant again. All of this made me wonder, what would my future look like if there were no children in it?

After wading through another panic attack at the mere thought of that possibility, I took several deep breaths and tried to construct that future. I have spent the last decade of my life planning my future to include a child. I have thought about schooling, immunizations, pediatricians, hobbies, etc. I don't have it all planned out, but I have had more time to think about these things than most parents do. It is hard to imagine a future life without a child in it.

Well, let's just say, I was unable to fill in the blank. At this point, everything else seems to pale in comparison to becoming a parent. I wouldn't put more effort into my work (I already do too much of that). I could start my own writing program (I will probably do that anyway), I could volunteer more (even though so much of my life revolves around helping others), and I could work on writing (I already do that).

I already have a great house, a good husband, two wonderful kitties, a job I love, etc. My life is pretty full, and yet why does it feel like a big chunk of it is missing?

Crash and Burn

April 25, 2010

IT WOULD APPEAR the period and the after effects of Clomid finally caught up with me, and I crashed hard this weekend. It started out with exhaustion on Friday, heavy flow on Saturday, and an enormous emotional meltdown today. All of this compounded by life's troubles: end of the semester craziness, a husband's gardening obsession, and my nephew's impending surgery.

My nephew Allen (the one with the ladybug) was born with a hole in his heart. Doctors implanted a pacemaker, and for the most part, it has been successful. He is a happy, extremely sensitive, little guy, and regular pacer checks showed for years that he was doing fine.

This past week, he ended up in the ER because his lead wire started to malfunction. They were considering doing emergency surgery, but decided to hold off until this coming Wednesday and replace the pacemaker entirely. I am scared for him, and he is scared for himself. He told his Dad, my brother, that he is afraid that he will die on the table. Such an emotional burden for a 13-year-old boy to bear! I would do anything to ease his fears.

Instead, his mother continues to deny our family contact with him. My parents and my brother plan on going to the hospital the day of his surgery. I will be there, too, but in the parking lot, waiting for word.

So, maybe when I broke down earlier this afternoon, it had more to do with my fear for my nephew's life than my own troubles. Whatever the source, I will be glad when this week has passed.

Wishing Well

April 29, 2010

"If you truly do not wish to, then you will not." –Ajahn Jumnian

TODAY'S WRITING comes out of several recent events. I wanted to wait until after my surgical consult this afternoon to post an entry, but said events seemed to call for a few lines.

Yesterday, my nephew had surgery to replace the battery and repair the lead wire in his pacemaker. Everything went well, and he is recovering just fine. Seeing him there in the bed, 13, fragile, yet strong with youth, I was overcome with deep anguish and joy. I held his hand as he struggled with what he called "loopiness," as the anesthesia wore off, and joked with him in a way that aunts do. Being there for him and my family was important to me even if it was incredibly painful.

Hospital waiting rooms give me flashbacks. The entire time I was waiting for word, my mind was on Nicholas. In one week of life, he had nine surgeries, thrice-daily blood transfusions, and innumerable other procedures. The sounds of beeping machines send me right back to those horrible days and nights that he struggled for life in the NICU. I was consoled only by the fact my nephew is strong and the doctors are well qualified. Of course, seeing him there weak in his bed made me wonder if having a child against all odds is worth it.

When we began this journey a few years ago, my husband and I talked about the risks involved. Given my history of child loss, he wondered if we would have to face such things together. He did not handle it well, saying at one point if I found myself standing over another baby's grave not to look to him for support. It would be my fault. Obviously, this did not go over too well with me, and I broke up with him for several months because of it.

Since then, we have had a few frank conversations about child loss. What do we do if we have a miscarriage or a child born dead? My answer is, and will always be, I don't know. Until such an horrendous moment happens, you have no idea how you will respond. It is a loss compared to no other. That's about all I can say. It is like wondering what would happen if I found out I had cancer. I have no idea how I would deal with that.

I think the question the husband was trying (okay, so he did it poorly) to ask is, is it worth the risk to get pregnant and then lose the child? My answer, of course, was developed through consultation with my doctors: yes. Because my previous losses were unrelated, there is no reason to expect that there will be more. Although having PCOS generally increases the potential for miscarriage, the factors involved are under control. Insulin resistance is one of them.

I opened this post with a quote about wishing. Rather, not wishing. I have wondered, as has my message lady, if perhaps because the losses have been so traumatic, somehow I am blocking myself from getting pregnant out of fear? Maybe, subconsciously, I am, but I don't think that is accurate. I am not sure why I have been unsuccessful up to this point, but I can say this for certain: it is not out of lack of support.

I have talked about the power of wishing, and the immense power of wishing for others. I truly believe that being involved in someone's wishing enterprise is essential to their wellbeing and your own. This concept was reiterated yesterday by two of my students.

It turns out that they have been reading my blog, which surprised me, because I am not sure I would be all that interested in my ramblings if I was a college freshman. I was deeply moved by their concern for me

They gave me an elephant keychain, which they said they saw on an Honors trip to Chicago and thought of me and my blog. Elephants, as you know, are good luck!

Recently I wondered what Samantha would be like today, at their age. I can only hope that she might have been like these two young women: kind, caring, smart, creative, and filled with passion for life. I would have been and am very proud!

They are wishing with me, as I know other readers are. I cannot thank you enough for that! Collective wishing must be more powerful than wishing alone.

Off to see the doctor. Pre-op consultation for the surgery on May 11. A post will no doubt be forthcoming.

The Dr. Made the Dr. Wait

April 29, 2010

MY FRIEND SAID the above after I got back from my pre-op appointment because I had to wait an hour, which meant I had to drive home in rush hour traffic. In the end, though, it was a good appointment. I learned quite a bit and feel better about what's going to happen on the day of the surgery.

He said I am not a good candidate for ovarian drilling because I respond to other treatments, like Clomid. What he will be doing in there is removing the blocked left tube, looking for and removing any adhesions, looking for and removing any endometriosis, and looking inside my uterus for any abnormalities. Hopefully, one of these strategies will work.

He did give me some positive feedback: that is good that I am 36 and not 40 and that I am in good health. He seemed hopeful, even if he was fairly brusque!

In any case, surgery is less than two weeks away. I will be glad when it is over.

May 2010

Facing the Unknown

May 1, 2010 at 7:20 am

ANOTHER RESTLESS NIGHT's sleep. I think that the anxiety about the upcoming surgery and the end-of-the-semester stress is hitting my sub-conscious (and now conscious) harder than I expected. Of course, I can't have any kind of surgery that requires total sedation without feeling a little panicked. It reminds me of when I nearly bled to death giving birth to Nicholas. And worst of all, his death.

About two months after he died, I had to have gallbladder surgery. It was in the same OR where he was born, and I absolutely went crazy. I could not go through with the surgery. I got right to the OR door, and freaked out. I pulled the IV out of my arm and ran out of the hospital (yeah, in the gown). I just did not want to die. It was overwhelming.

Two weeks after that, I had the surgery, but only after they injected me with the absolute maximum dose of sedation! In addition, my favorite priest came to sit with me. He was an incredible comfort. Sigh.

Now, in a little over a week, I am going to face that scenario again. I have absolute confidence in my doctor. Despite his cockiness, I know that he knows what he is doing. He has done several surgeries just like this over many years and was just voted one of the best doctors in Pittsburgh.

And yet . . . we all know that things go wrong. He pointed them out, of course. And it is these unknown variables that scare me.

Worst of all is the unknown husband factor. He has said he is still not sure he can take the day off. I thought about just having my parents go, but they won't drive to the city. My girlfriends live pretty far away. (One of them is coming up the week after the surgery.) So I wonder, am I going to get stuck in Pittsburgh and not be able to make it home on the day I have surgery? If that happens, I plan on just staying the night at the hotel next door.

It is times like these that I feel abandoned, I guess.

And then there is the fact that if he does show up will he be of any comfort at all? I mean, I want someone there who will be more than just a ride, but a support person as well. I could get some very bad news. I guess only time will tell what happens.

I do wonder what I will do if he doesn't show up . . .

Wishes–They Come True in Pairs

May 3, 2010 at 11:22 pm

I HAVE MENTIONED BEFORE about my estranged relationship with my beloved nephews. I have spent the last three years of my life dealing with their mother, who dangles them in front of me and my family like meat before a dog. She will let me talk to them on the phone in the morning and ban me from their lives later that day.

But recently things have changed. I got to see my youngest nephew on his birthday and when he had surgery. Then, I got to see my oldest nephew, too. I found out today that he is going to be staying with my brother for at least a couple of weeks, which means I will get to see him more often!

Of course, all of this makes me wonder if my original suppositions were correct. Every time I have had my fortune told, the teller has always said that I would have two children. I have always believed that those kids were not my own but my nephews. They always said no; the children are mine.

In any case, I am hopeful that I will be able to spend time with them this summer. I need them in my life.

Ironic, No?

May 8, 2010 at 3:26 pm

AND ALL OF THIS TIME I have been trying to get pregnant, and now I find myself in an odd position. It turns out that I ovulated about a week earlier than usual. Of course, I was not abstaining from sex because I had no idea that I would ovulate on day 10!!

Now, I am worried that that the blood work coming up before the surgery will not be accurate to determine whether we conceived or not. It confuses me because the doctor said that it should be accurate, but how can that be given that the a fertilized egg doesn't even implant for 6-12 days after fertilization. I am concerned to say the least. I find myself fearing that I am pregnant!

In any case, the doctor will be doing blood work on Monday and then I will take a home pg test when I get up on the day of surgery. I sure hope that if I did manage to get pregnant (unlikely) that one of the tests will pick it up.

On Mothers and Mother's Day

May 8, 2010 at 5:03 pm

SAMANTHA WAS MURDERED in November 1991. My very first Mother's Day following her death, my neighbor leaned out her kitchen door and shouted a cheery "Happy Mother's Day!" It was crushing. She did not mean to hurt my feelings, but I wore that sadness around my neck like a too-tight scarf for the rest of that day.

Since then, I have weathered many Mother's Days relatively well. I don't really get all that upset. After all, I get to celebrate with my own mother. It is surprising to me that it is not more difficult for me to endure, but I think because my children died so young, long before they could understand a commercialized day such as this one, that I guess I just don't miss what I never had.

To celebrate the day, I took a trip out to where I was born yesterday. I hadn't been to Loudenville, West Virginia since I was maybe eight years old, so I wasn't sure what I would find. Rather, I wasn't sure what I would think of the place where I spent all nine of my prenatal months and the first six months of my life outside the womb. It was a fitting journey for Mother's Day since my Mom and I had to fend for ourselves those long months, and it really was a fight for survival.

You won't find Loudenville on most maps. It isn't even listed on epodunk.com. The most information that can be found online about this community located in rural Marshall County is its longitude, latitude, and elevation. Basically, you can find Loudenville if you take 88-S for a bit, then 250 for a bit, then some back roads. It is not far from Cameron or Glen Easton, which are not large towns by any means.

The drive was a good one. It was 80 degrees and I was on the back of my husband's bike. I intended to go alone, but he offered, and I have a hard time resisting a motorcycle ride, especially out in the West Virginia (and yes, it is a state) countryside. It is one of the reasons I moved back. The smell of spring flowers, fresh cut grass, and hay. West Virginia really is almost Heaven!

As we drove on through the warm May sunshine, the stories of my first few months of life roared through my mind as loudly as the engine. My mother said when she brought me home from the hospital on Halloween in 1973, she placed me in a basinet in the corner of the small room we shared with her grandmother. The three of us lived in an abandoned church right before the bridge in Loudenville.

My father abandoned my mother when she found out she was pregnant. (When I met him at age 13, he claimed to not know that I existed, even though his brother was married to my Mom's sister. Um, yeah.) My mother had dropped out of school in the eighth grade and had no real marketable skills. She had worked, briefly, in the garment district in New York and as a dish washer in Brown's Restaurant in Cameron, but there was little suitable work for a pregnant woman in rural West Virginia.

We survived, according to my mother, on $17 a month in food stamps and wild game and garden vegetables that were dropped off at their door step by family members. It was a hard time for all of us. During her pregnancy, my mother says she was limited to potatoes for nearly every meal. It is no wonder, then, that few people could tell for sure if she was pregnant even up to the day before I was born. I weighed 6 lbs and 2 oz.

My mother also told me that the heat in the little church would go out in the winter, forcing us to flee to the neighbor's house in the night. Snow would come into the window and onto my basinet. It was a rough place to live.

Knowing all of this, I was not surprised at all when we pulled up to a falling-over house to confirm that we had indeed found Loudenville. The young woman sitting on her porch happily nodded as her two small children and many orange tabby cats approached our bike. Her partner appeared from under the hood of a car and gave us directions back to the main road.

She asked who we were looking for, and I said no one. "I was born here, and just wanted to visit." She smiled. I smiled back. And we drove away.

On the way back, I sighed, thinking about those early days. I had always been so proud of myself for having pulled myself up by my bootstraps and somehow managed to get out of abject poverty and into a comfortable lifestyle with a doctoral education. But that day, I struggled with that notion. I began to question my own self narrative. In the light of that warm Friday evening, I saw for the first time that I did overcome a lot, but there is no shame in the place where I am from.

No, I would not want to live there now. I love where I live. I like being close to stores, the library, and other places that are important to me. And yet there is a simple beauty to this place from whence I came. Green trees for miles. Fields of wild flowers. A rolling creek.

At the same time, I know that my mother was terribly unhappy there. She couldn't even afford to buy maxi-pads. She had no privacy. She struggled with the small-minded views of the people in the tiny community.

On the way back home, we took, in a sense, my life path. From Loudenville to Moundsville to Wheeling. There were pitstops along the way: a few months in Powhatan Point, Ohio, a few more in Proctor, WV, seven years in Athens, Ohio, five years in Cincinnati, Ohio, and one year in California, Pennsylvania. But no life is linear. And my reflections on my life aren't either.

As soon as I got home, I called my mother. She talked to me about where I had been, explaining to me what I had seen. Like so many other parts of my life, I need her to put moments and places into a context, so I can understand.

It makes me wonder what kind of stories I will tell my children. Will I take them to this place where my life began? Will I teach them to respect the world that we are from? Or will I use it as it has been used for me, as a lesson of how not to live your life? As a warning? Or will I choose to explain more as I see it now, as the place where I managed to survive amid the hazards of cold and near starvation? Not as a warning but as a tale of endurance and possibility.

Pre-Op Post

May 10, 2010

Surgery in the early, early am. Laproscopic. Worried about the outcome. Will post more post-op.

A Post-Op Post

May 11, 2010

The surgery was about ten hours ago. I am at home recovering. Eating saltines, drinking tea, and looking forward to a nice long nap.

It was scary. I guess any time general anesthesia is administered it is dangerous. I was able to hold on for most of the time. I didn't really start to get panicky until about 10 minutes before show time.

I woke up with a terrible headache and a bit of pain, but otherwise, I am doing just fine.

My husband came through like a real champ. I couldn't have asked for a better support person. I was impressed and quite thankful for him. He stayed with me through all of it and started crying when he finally got to see me in recovery. He was scared because it took a little longer than predicted. I am glad my fears about his role in all of this were not justified.

I did not get to talk to the doctor, but this is what he told the husband. He removed the bad left fallopian tube, some scar tissue near it, and scar tissue in my uterus from the placental abruption. The right side is great. He told hubby there is no reason I cannot have a successful pregnancy. Now, we just have to do it!

Sitting on the couch reading and enjoying some movies is not a bad way to begin my first week of summer break. Too bad I had to have surgery to earn it!

Recovering in the Garden

May 14, 2010

IT HAS BEEN FOUR DAYS since the surgery, and I am feeling better. Although I am taking it easy, I can't help but wander out into the garden to see how my sprouts are doing. They are growing so quickly, and it has made me ponder what my life will be like when I pick the first tomato or slice up the first cucumber. Will I be on fertility drugs? Will I be pregnant? Will I be going to IVF classes? Maybe we will be out sailing!

In any case, I recall what my husband said the day before my surgery: "Tomorrow will be the beginning for us." He meant that we will be preparing ourselves for IVF this summer. And I think in many ways he is right. The doctor gave us a clean bill of health, so to speak, and we are ready to get to work.

At the same time, I feel like I have put quite a bit of work into this process already. And in some ways, I am tired. Not just from the surgery, but from trying too hard. We have spent the first year of our marriage trying to get pregnant, which has been incredibly stressful.

In any case, every morning I wake up and look at the garden and get excited about what the future holds. With the hope that the deer don't find my garden until I get the fence up!

Contemplating Futures

May 15, 2010

I REALIZED THIS AFTERNOON that if I get pregnant this year or next, then I will have given birth once a decade: 1991, 2001, and then 2011. Since those children also died the same year that they were born, I am more than a little apprehensive about it. Of course, I realize this is destructive thinking. After all, there is no guarantee I will get pregnant.

Sadly, this point was brought to my attention this afternoon when my husband said, "I really don't think we will have children." He has said this all along, though I had hoped that my surgery (just four short days ago) would have changed his mind. He said it proves nothing to him. He has given up on ever being a father.

Perhaps I am risking a complete mental collapse here, but I just can't be that pessimistic. Even on my darkest days (right around my period, for example), I do not give up all hope of having a child. He has resigned himself (and me, in his own way) to being a perpetual empty nester. I asked him why my doctor's post-op comments about improving my fertility through the surgery did not buoy his hopes. He said, "Nothing's changed. It is just not meant to be."

It is crushing when one half of the partnership feels a project is doomed from the start, but I guess I just have to double my wishes to compensate.

At the same time, we spend countless hours discussing parenting styles and what we think we will be like as parents. Admittedly, this is most assuredly putting the horse before the old chariot. Expending mental energy on something that may not come to pass is really not productive nor fair to my already troubled mind.

Of course, I am not one to let that stop me.

I just finished reading *Beauty Before Comfort*, a memoir/biography by Allison Glock. I was drawn to the book because it was: 1. written by a woman from northern Appalachia, specifically WV, 2. a memoir, 3. just a buck at the library book sale. It is a complicated narrative about the author's grandmother, who was the belle of Chester/Newell, WV (famous for Homer Laughlin pottery...Fiesta Ware to you).

Given that motherhood is on my mind, I read this book as a study in parenting, as much as a historical piece about my home state. I was simultaneously appalled and enthralled by Glock's recollections of her childhood and her grandmother's childhood. Angered at the capacity for cruelty that some parents can have and moved by the personal defeat that often leads them to those dark places and behaviors. As I read I was very aware of how hurt is passed on from one generation to the next like heart disease and alcoholism.

I have my share of mental troubles. I have been diagnosed with generalized anxiety disorder, post-traumatic stress disorder, and more recently, co-dependency. None of these are life threatening conditions, but they sure threaten my quality of life. And I don't want my children to inherit them by blood or by deed.

These concerns have been cemented by other recent readings, including my latest memoir, *Searching for Mercy Street*, Linda Gray Sexton. She is the daughter of the wonderful, tragic poet, Anne Sexton. Here is one of the poems by Anne that I remember most:

I Remember

I am only halfway through the book, but it has been illuminating. Sadly, I am seeing in myself many of the behaviors and moods that Anne Sexton exhibited, which is not good. She ended up committing suicide after several attempts over many decades. I am not suicidal, but I do have dark depressions and I do act out those crushing moods in childish ways sometimes. I guess comparing myself to her is unfair, especially given that she was completely off the deep end for quite some time.

Nonetheless, seeing what her behavior did to her children has reinforced in me the need to be the best person I can be to be the best parent I can be.

Linda Gray Sexton's tale reinforces my notion that bad parenting can be overcome. Maybe not completely, but if we try and we are aware, then surely we can do better than our parents did for us. Surely, I can give my kids more than my parents gave to me.

Searching for Help

May 19, 2010

IF YOU HAVE BEEN reading along, then you know I have been under stress. Yeah, I know, who wouldn't be given the fertility drugs, surgery, LIFE? But reading the auto/biography of Anne Sexton really put my concerns in my face. Throughout her daughter Linda's book I was struck by just how hard it is to break the patterns of the past.

What I didn't expect was that Linda would have so many struggles with infertility in her own life! It turns out that Anne began bleeding early into her pregnancy and a doctor gave her DES, which the world later discovered caused high rates of vaginal and cervical cancer later in the children's lives. Sadly, many women whose mother's took DES later found out that they were infertile due in part by malformed uteruses. Linda is one of those women.

Nonetheless, after being told that she would never have children, she discovered that she was pregnant and went on to have two healthy boys. It gave me hope, which was immediately dashed by her revelations that her own parenting practices were haunted by the ghost of her mother.

She found herself screaming at her children and unable to calm down. She felt as though she no longer wanted to be a mother. She even spanked her children when she really knew that was not how she wanted to parent. I was stunned. I thought for sure that she was so aware; aware enough to parent in a healthy way. Eventually, she went to therapy and even began taking an anti-depressant to treat what she realized was an inherited mental condition. She ends the book asserting that she finally got a handle on her unproductive behaviors and became a better parent.

Friday Night Blues—Remix

May 21, 2010

I KNOW THAT MANY of my recent posts have not been all that chipper. Ever since my illness a few months ago, I have struggled to find that happy spot that allowed me to believe that my wish–to have a healthy child–would come true. I can feel that light building again, so if you are praying and wishing for me, keep it up! I can feel the difference.

I had a great day today. I spent around twelve hours with my best friend, who moved away several years ago. We did the silly things we always do: lunch, shop, chat. Then, I invited a few people over for an impromptu gathering on my deck. It is a nice summer evening, and it is hard to resist spending some of that time outdoors. As my guests were leaving, I pulled my best friend aside and said to her, "I have a good life." And for the first time in a long time I meant it. More importantly, I felt it.

I wonder, then, how do the sad moods keep me down? How do I get so far down that I feel like I will never get back up?

Lately, I have been trying to document my moods to leave a record to show myself that I do get depressed but I do come out of it. In the first picture I took, I am suffering mightily. I felt out of control, abandoned, rejected, and hopeless.

And in one taken just three days later, while in the company of my best friend, I am incredibly happy once again. I do seem to do better around others, but I don't think that can be the only reason my mood turned around.

It is almost like I am a different person.

I don't expect every day to be wonderful. In fact, I don't expect to be happy all day every day, but I am starting to get the idea that there can be happiness found in each day if only I look for it.

All the Truth That's Fit to Blog

May 26, 2010

LATELY, I HAVE BEEN pondering memory quite a bit more than usual. My training in creative non-fiction was really my first introduction to theorizing memory and truth and fact. Up to that point (maybe a decade ago), I knew that everyone had different memories of the same event, but I always assumed that my version was the TRUE version and they must have misremembered.

My husband and I talked about truth and memory today as we took the motorcycle to a lake about an hour away. He remembered quite clearly he used to go there as a child. He told me all about the fishing and swimming he used to do there with his brothers and sisters and how much fun he had with the other teens that stayed there in the summer. His memories seemed precise, including details of the cottage where they stayed several times.

When we got to the marina, he exclaimed, "Wow. That is much smaller than I remember! When I was a kid, the lake seemed so vast."

We then talked about faulty or incomplete memories over lunch, which is a common conversation for us. We have both learned that while our memories might be important to us, they are not fact but an impression that can be shaped over time by new experiences and forgetfulness.

I will save my theoretical discussion of truth and memory for another entry, but I think it is important to give a nod to truth here. As many of you know, I am pretty frank about my life, my feelings, my thoughts, my experiences. I intend to be. Therefore, I can tell you, faithful readers, that I endeavor to tell the truth as I know it. And if I should question that truth, whether it be memory or fact, I will do it willingly and out in the open for all to read. Truth can, after all, set a person free.

In other news, I see the doctor tomorrow for my post-op appointment, and I expect him to tell me the truth: Have my chances of conception increased after the operation? Should I try a few more times with Clomid to get pregnant before moving on to IVF? I hope he can be honest and his own desire to profit from IVF does not cloud his judgment or his advice.

I am nervous about this appointment. Even though my husband assures me the doctor told him everything went well and my right tube and ovary are perfect, I fear that my husband misunderstood him or didn't quite hear what he said. I suppose that is just my anxiety working against me. I will post about the follow up as soon as I can.

In future entries, a discussion of "secondary victimization." Yeah, chew on that for a bit.

A Post-Post-Op Post

May 27, 2010

NOW THAT YOU HAVE untangled the title of this post, settle in for a bit of doctor speak. I will try to decode it as best I can.

I had my surgery follow-up appointment yesterday afternoon, and I learned much about what he found during the surgery. My husband's explanation was actually fairly simplistic, but I am thinking that is because he did not get the full story.

The doctor did remove my left fallopian tube. It was swollen (hydrosalpinx) and blocked. He removed the adhesions where it was attached to my bowel. My husband had said that there was scar tissue in my uterus. There was not. Instead, the doctor discovered that my uterus is fluffy.

That's right boys and girls, the actual medical term is "fluffy." According to my research, a fluffy uterus is a good thing in some ways because it demonstrates a full, plush uterine lining, which is good for fetus implantation. On the other hand, it can conceal endometrial polyps.

Basically, an endometrial polyp looks like a little tree with branches and nodules. The polyp itself is usually about the size of a pencil eraser. Most polyps are noncancerous, but they can cause spotting and even miscarriages. They are difficult to remove during a D&C because they can be pushed back by the scalpel, so they are typically removed during a hysterscopy, which is one of the procedures I had done.

I mention all of this because he found what he thinks was an endometrial polyp. He sent it out for testing, and it came back benign as did the swollen left tube and my endometrial tissue. So, the good news is that I am cancer free. The bad news is the dye he inserted into my right tube did not spill back out.

When he told me that there could be a blockage in my right tube I wanted to cry, but instead I listened to what he had to say instead of allowing my mind to make the worst of an unknown situation. I have a bad habit of doing that and I often learn less because of it. He explained he thinks it is extremely unlikely that the tube is actually blocked. There are no medical reasons for why it would be and there are other reasons for why that dye did not spill back out, including gravity!

To make absolutely sure that it is open, he has ordered me to have another hystersalpingogram (HSG), which is a painful and challenging procedure. Basically, I get up on this five-foot tall table, put my legs behind my head (not an exaggeration), and the technician shoots dye into my uterus and up into my tubes to see if the tubes are open. Lefty was closed, but righty has always been open, so hopefully that is what this test will confirm.

I left the office with mixed emotions. On the one hand, I was glad I didn't have cancer or some other type of serious disease, such as Asherman's Syndrome (webbing in the uterus). On the other hand, the thought of having a blocked right tube just threw me. If that tube is blocked, there will be no babies through natural conception, ever. And the idea of another procedure! I wanted to give up right then and there. No more procedures! No more trying!

I allowed my mind to focus on the doom and gloom for about 15 minutes, then I snapped out of it. I considered the following: he said it was extremely unlikely for that tube to actually be blocked and even if it is, we can still have a baby through IVF. Tubes are not required. Also, he did say my ovaries looked very healthy as did my uterus. I know for a fact the news could have been direr. I must focus on the good.

I asked if we should consider doing a few more rounds of Clomid since the problems he corrected were more than likely preventing conception. He said we could do that. After the HSG, I will make a decision about what to do next: more Clomid or on to IVF.

If I had money and didn't have a job, I would do IVF immediately. It is very costly (around 20K) and it is extremely hard on the body and mind. My husband and I have accepted that we will likely have to turn to IVF, so we are prepared for it financially, but who wants to spend that kind of money if you don't have to?

Now, I wait. My period has been delayed by the surgery, but as soon as it starts, I will make an appointment for the HSG. After the results come back, I will talk to my doctor about our next step. Meanwhile, I will enjoy my summer without the pressure of timed intercourse or taking my temperature or charting my cervical mucus. I will sit on my back deck and enjoy the sunset and have quiet dinners with my husband. I have accepted there is nothing easy about this journey I have chosen to take, but I do know I can step off the path any time.

Presumptuous Watermelon Vines

May 28, 2010

IN REALITY, the watermelon vines were not the presumptuous ones—we were. When I was around four years old, my Dad's factory went on strike for more than a year, and we lost our house. We had to move into a trailer, but my parents believed that it would only be temporary. Temporary turned out to be 19 years, but I digress.

When I was in eighth grade, my parents were offered a house to rent by our landlord. A house! If you have ever spent the night in a 60s-era, single-wide trailer, you know there is quite a bit of difference between mobile home living and living in a house. In a house the walls don't shake when your Dad gets out of bed or when the wind blows hard. In a house your bathwater doesn't get cold before you finish filling the tub because there is no insulation and no foundation. Perhaps more importantly, it would be far harder for someone to haul your house away, but a truck could drag a MOBILE home to the other side of town with not much more effort than a wide load sticker.

Perhaps I have simplified and even demonized trailer park living, but I can tell you that it was not the best place to grow up. And not the worst place either!

When we learned that the landlord had a house available, my brother, mother, dad, and grandma (who lived with us) began packing immediately. Oddly enough, the first items we moved were the contents of our cupboards: canned food, macaroni, rice, taco shells. I remember in a fuzzy sort of way unloading those non-perishable items onto the pantry shelves in the new place. It wasn't a mansion by any means, but it had a firmly attached porch that didn't rock when you stepped on it and it had a second floor.

Earlier that summer, we had planted watermelon seeds in front of the trailer. They were from a store-bought melon, so none of us thought that anything would become of them. We were all surprised when a little sprout appeared, followed by a vine, and then a green piece of fruit that looked like a miniature Zeppelin. When we were assured the house was ours to rent, we pondered the fate of that extraordinary plant. It was decided that we chop it down because we didn't want the next family to enjoy the literal fruits of our labor.

I can still see my brother, butcher knife in hand, hacking at that struggling plant and then tearing it by the root from the arid soil. It seemed an extreme act to me then, but even more so now. I think our attitude then had to do with the bitterness that had built from living all those years in the trailer court. Our neighbors had gone from working class stiffs like my dad to people barely getting by on public assistance. People came and went and with them alcohol and violence.

Not long after our watermelon friend met his end, our landlord informed us he had sold the house. We would have to stay in the trailer. He had no other houses available. At the time, this turn of fate seemed almost expected. After all, as my mother still says, "You just can't get ahead." We retrieved our canned corn and dried beans and filled in the hole where the watermelon plant once grew. And life went back to what it was before: hot (no air conditioning) and chaotic.

These memories came to me while I was in the garden today. It is far different than that little, dusty patch in front of the trailer. But I didn't dwell on the physical contrast between the two. Rather, I wondered why we would make such a seemingly mean-spirited choice. Why cut down the watermelon vine so that the next tenants couldn't have it? What does this say about our mindsets then? What does it say about my mindset now? I could have understood transplanting the watermelon to the next location, but destroying it for others seems immature and vengeful.

I suppose it was a symbolic act, which destroyed any connection we had to the trailer and the trailer court, but even if we had not returned to that place, the impression would have remained. Perhaps it was our way of acting out our discomfort with calling some other place home. As much as we disliked living in the trailer court, it was where we lived.

Soren Kierkegaard writes, "Life can only be understood backwards, but it must be lived forwards." I think today's post is about looking back, so that I can live on. I recoil from the memory of my brother's arm swinging the knife like a machete and seeing the just-growing fruit tossed into the gravel road that ran too close to our front steps. I have held onto this memory because I want to remember not to hate the next person that comes along. I want to remember sometimes change can hurt, but there is no reason to destroy the past.

I look now at a summer of uncertainty, but I suppose the future is always uncertain. Normally, that would scare me. My life has taught me the more out of control I feel, the more in control I try to be. I realize control is impossible. Things happen. Life happens. I am getting better at accepting that reality, but instead of dreading it, I am looking towards the future hopefully. Whatever happens, happens.

After all, as David Copper says in *The Heart of Stillness*, "The unknown is a territory where truth is hidden." I think I will wander off into the unknown awhile. Perhaps I will find the truth behind the destruction of those watermelon vines.

(In)decisions

May 31, 2010

I SUPPOSE, really, that no concrete decision has been made, but we did have a talk about the IVF situation. Oddly enough, a discussion about buying a boat brought it on.

We have been talking about renting a boat and sailing it on the ocean since around Christmas time, and then the other day, we decided we were going to buy a row boat so we could enjoy some time sailing around here. We both like to be on the water, and buying a boat seems like a good idea. We even found one on sale the other day, after looking at over eight sporting goods stores. We didn't buy the boat because we were on the motorcycle and had no way to transport it. We plan on buying it this coming weekend and dragging it home on the roof of his car.

Of course, the decision to buy the row boat came after a lengthy discussion about our proposed sailing trip. Can we feasibly do both of those things AND IVF in the same summer? We came to the conclusion that no, we cannot.

After hashing it out over some grilled Tofurkey sausages and some work in the garden, we concluded that we would find out the results of the upcoming HSG before making a final decision. If the right tube is not blocked (we are pretty sure that it is not), then we will do a few more cycles of Clomid. My thinking is that if the issues we corrected during surgery were enough to prevent implantation or cause miscarriage, then why not give Clomid another try? The idea of something more drastic than Clomid just seems untenable at the moment. We will then defer IVF until next summer.

If the tube is blocked, then we will do IVF as early as December.

At the time of the conversation, I hesitantly agreed to this plan. Now, it scares me. By this time next year, I will be 37 pushing 38. So many months...12...will have gone by. Can I cope for another year?

The pros of waiting are we can save more money, our marriage will be even stronger, and I should be even healthier. The cons are as I age the risks of miscarriage, birth defects, and many other problems increase dramatically. As I sit here now, two rooms away from my husband, able to see only by the glow of my monitor screen and keyboard lights, I feel like shouting, "We have to do it now!"

I am glad the pressure is temporarily off in terms of us having a baby. We are both more relaxed. But in the back of my mind, the nagging voices of future concern and possible regret have grown a little louder.

At one point today (and at several points earlier this week), I was ready to walk away from trying altogether. I was ready to say, if it happens, it does. If it doesn't, it doesn't. Of course, that has never been my way of navigating life. If I want something, I tend to pursue it doggedly. At the same time, I was so happy with how life was going. We spent the weekend playing together: riding the motorcycle, dreaming about boating and fishing, making love, watching movies, just enjoying each other's company. And during the entire weekend, I kept thinking: I can live like this. I can enjoy being with this person in this way in our lovely home for the rest of my life. Children would be wonderful, but I can live without them. My life is full and joyous. I have great friends, jobs I love, and overall, good health.

Then, the call came.

At first I didn't realize this is what had changed my perspective. Not until I got halfway through this entry did I realize my thoughts about having children or not have been influenced by the death of my husband's uncle. The call came in this afternoon while we were riding on the bike on the back roads above the river. We stopped so that he could talk.

He hasn't seen that side of his family in nearly twenty years, but, of course, the pain of the loss is still real. He then began talking to me about his family, cousins, aunts, other uncles, and how much he was looking forward to seeing them, even under such sad conditions. Then, he began talking about how their children must have grown. How that will be the talk of the evening: children. And I found myself longing, once again, to be part of that conversation.

So often I feel left out when people talk about their children, but only because I, too, have children stories. My kids didn't live long, but I have great memories of them that I feel compelled to share but so often don't, out of fear of making others feel uncomfortable.

He then told me he wanted to go to the viewing alone but I could come to the funeral if I wanted to. I felt hurt, even though I know that I shouldn't. We all deal with loss in different ways. If he doesn't want me there, it is for a reason, but I have to wonder if it is in part because he thinks I will be uncomfortable about all this chatter of children. At the same time, I think he will find he misses me. I have been in his life for nearly 17 years. There have been ups and downs, but I have been there. And now I am his wife. Nonetheless, I will support him in the way he wishes, even if it means I have to do that from afar. I have to remind myself this is his loss, not mine.

I hope when the time comes that we do attempt IVF we can be on the same page on what the other person needs. It will be an incredibly hard time for me, emotionally and physically. I will need his support more than ever. He will need my support, too, but it seems that we often mistake our own needs for the needs of others. Earlier he said that we often underestimate each other and what we need. I disagree. I know he is strong, but I also know a hand to hold in a time of grief is usually more help than harm.

Throughout this day of great decisions, I have walked away more uncertain than ever. Is it too risky to wait to do IVF? Should I go to the viewing with him anyway because I anticipate he will need me more than he realizes? Or should I just get in that row boat and ride out the waves? I suppose I have answered my own questions. I need to just roll with the tide. Otherwise, I will eat away at my own happiness, which defeats the point of living my best life.

June 2010

Letting Go

June 2, 2010

ONE OF THE MAIN tenets of the Al-Anon program is, "let go and let God." I understand this to mean that you have to let go of whatever it is that is bothering you and let God take the burden from your heart. I have never been good at that. I overanalyze and beat to death just about anything that puzzles or hurts me. I twist it, shake it, and bend it. Of course, few good things come of that. While those strategies might work for me as a writer and as a reader of texts, they don't work for me in my personal life. Such obsessive thinking leads only to sadness and even more frustration.

I know, however, that letting go of something is just as important as striving for others. I just sometimes get the two mixed up.

Our culture rewards our tenacity, our never-give-up mentality. But rarely is the strength it takes to let go ever recognized. Therefore, we just don't learn it. We become masters of never letting things rest. Like The Beatles said so long ago, "Let it be."

My struggles with letting go are multiple, but the one I work so hard on is motherhood, but I have made great progress recently. I am in the process of letting it go.

For twenty years I have tried to be a mother. That role has been stripped of me four times through murder, premature birth, ectopic pregnancy, and blighted ovum. And now a fifth time by my own hand. I spent my money for IVF to buy a house. I guess I assumed at the time it was important to have a home and I would make the money back in no time. But that hasn't happened. In an effort to spend more time with my husband and just enjoy my life, I have cut back on work (my second job), and my bank accounts are not where they were a year ago.

Of course, there is no guarantee IVF would even work, but I threw away my chances of even trying anytime in the near future when I bought this house. And I love my house.

Yes, Clomid could work or even trying on our own now that I have had the surgery, but I really feel like I am done trying. The anxiety of taking my temperature daily, checking my cervical mucus, keeping track of when we have sex, and all of the other minute and mundane rituals involved in this quest seem untenable. I mean, it's been twenty years!

Beyond that, I am 36 now. Do I want to wake up at 3 am for diaper changes and feedings? Can I handle those tasks, and do them well, and still do my job?

The idea of giving up now after all this makes me feel sad, but years ago I promised myself I would stop trying at 35. After 35 the rates of Downs Syndrome, miscarriage, and pre-term birth escalate.

More than anything else, though, I am tired of living my life waiting. I feel like I have spent the better part of the last twenty years caught in between places, but never really anywhere. I was either pregnant, trying to get pregnant, waiting to try and get pregnant, or grieving over child loss. There hasn't been a time since 1990 that motherhood and its potential haven't overshadowed my daily living. I haven't really been living in the present, but only in the past and in the future, and I think it is time all of that stops.

Furthermore, I have realized one of the reasons why I have been so set on having a baby, when I had all but given up the quest with my ex-husband, is I want to have my husband's child because I think it might make him love me more. I know that it may sound crazy, but a year or two ago, he said I was not special, no better than any other woman he had dated. I suppose I get what he was saying in a practical sense, but in an emotional one, I was dumbstruck. Since then, I have seen how he is when he sees a Mom and her child. I just want him to look at me like that. Like I am special because I am the mother of his child.

Of course, this is not the ONLY reason I wished for children. There are so many other reasons, including those I don't understand and cannot articulate.

All of that said, I am preparing myself for letting go. In a sense, I am choosing to be child-free before that option is chosen for me. It will take so much strength to let go, and I even hear that voice in my head saying, "Just try one more cycle." And I want to silence that voice. I need to let go of this obsession and enjoy my life.

I am finally married to the love of my life. So many twists and turns brought us here, 17 years after we met. My marriage should be my top priority (after me, of course), but I have let it go aground more times than I can count because of my desire to have a child. I cannot abide by that any longer.

So, how will I do it? Make a list of all of the things I will do now that I am not trying to get pregnant and not planning to share my life with a child. Focus my energies on other, equally important things. But diversions are merely the beginning. The hardest part, even harder than letting go, is grieving. Grieving for the life that will never be. Grieving for the life I have dreamed about for two decades. Imaging a new future for myself absent of a child.

I begin with my list of things I can do if there will be no children:

1. Travel abroad. I can earn a Fulbright Scholarship and teach in a foreign country. I get paid from my school and from the government.
2. Work on my music. I am a singer and a song writer. Years ago I dreamed of making a CD of duets with all of my friends. It wouldn't be for money, but for the beauty of friendship and music making.

3. Buy a cabin in the mountains of West Virginia. We have talked about this extensively in recent months. We could buy a little cabin that we could use as a refuge, a place where we could go to enjoy fishing and hiking and boating and get away from it all for a while.
4. Volunteer at a cat shelter. I am allergic to cats. Hard to believe, I know, given that I love cats more than any other being (including people). I have two, and that is enough in terms of allergy problems. I have avoided volunteering at a shelter because of the inflammation that comes with allergy attacks is not good during conception or pregnancy.
5. Get a second PhD. I have been looking into a PhD program in Clinical Psychology. It would be a free degree, and I could use it to get into consulting. I want to look at the relationship between writing and mental health.
6. Get in shape. Yes, I can do that whether I am trying to get pregnant or not, but I have to be careful when TTC. I can't lift too much, I can't allow my body to get overheated, and I must avoid exercise that causes too much strain. All of these things can cause miscarriage or no implantation.
7. Stop taking Glucophage. This medication is dreadful. It causes upset stomach and vitamin B deficiency. I take it for PCOS, but mostly to get pregnant and prevent miscarriage, but if I am not trying to have a baby, I am going off of it and finding a more natural way of treating PCOS.
8. Take anti-depressants. I can't take them if I am trying to get pregnant. The risk of birth defects and other problems are just far too high. But in the absence of a potential pregnancy, I can maybe get a hold of my sometimes out of control emotions.
9. Spend more time writing. All of the time I spent researching spotting and implantation and early pregnancy signs and all of the other questions I have while trying to get pregnant could be used to work on the projects that always seem to get left behind. No more!

10. Work on being the best person possible. In absence of the TTC stress, I can work on being a better person overall, especially being a better wife.

This is just a partial list. The beginning of things to come; a life to unfold.

What will it feel like for that weight to be lifted? For the longing in my heart to be replaced with new life experiences instead of anticipation and anxiety?

My first step is to walk a labyrinth. There are several nearby. The walking around and around and around the path will be soothing and will help me better understand my decision, and I hope, it will help me let go.

Changes Come

June 4, 2010

THE TITLE REFERS to a song by Over the Rhine, my favorite band. The founding members, Karin and Linford (husband and wife) grew up not far from me on the Ohio side of the river, so that makes their music resonate with me all the more. "Changes Come" is about what you might think. Karin sings in the chorus:

> *Changes come*
> *Turn my world around*
> *Changes come*
> *Bring the whole thing down*

So much of my life in the last year has been about change. I moved back to the Ohio Valley, I bought a house, I got married. The changes have been difficult in some ways but more than worth the effort. But sometimes changes that turn my world around can also bring the whole thing down.

Two-Week Wait

We went to my husband's uncle's funeral today. It was incredibly moving, and I cried throughout the ceremony. Even though I didn't know this part of his family, their loss was crushing and their eulogies were heartfelt. As each child read a letter to their now deceased father, I was struck by thoughts of my own fathers (a biological father and a step-dad who raised me from three months on), my husband's father (he passed away a few years before I met my husband), and the fact that my husband will probably never be a father. I know this is something he wants, and it hurts me that I can't give him a child.

At dinner tonight he said he was thinking similar thoughts during the service and he realized his name will die with him. It is tough to be in this spot. Wanting so much to have a child with him but knowing I have reached my limit when it comes to fertility treatments. He thinks I will change my mind in the future and that might happen, but at this point, I just need to be free of it. I spent some time this afternoon reading stories from women who were or are in the same situation: the baby quest is ruining our lives.

But changes come. People die. Others are born. One minute you can be riding on the back of a motorcycle reveling in your good fortune and the next minute you discover a beloved family member is dead.

I have never believed that things happen for a reason. I see no sense in global hunger, the oil spill in the Gulf, my children's deaths. I believe changes come, whether we want them to or not. It is our job to figure out how to respond to those changes. We must choose how to live our lives in the best possible way knowing we have no control over what will happen next, which is one of the most difficult tasks I face.

Growing up in a household with an out of control father, I quickly learned how to attain the appearance of control. As an adult, I have realized trying to control my life is more harmful than good. But learning how to live that realization is going to be hardest part. I am reminded of a Tibetan Proverb:

> *You cannot discover new oceans unless you have the courage to lose sight of the shore.*

I must lose sight of the shore. I must not allow this fertility battle to control me any longer. I cannot cling to it and use it as a crutch to ignore the other wonderful things in my life.

Yes, I would love to be a mother, but I understand more and more every day that I need to let go. I must live my life instead of letting my life live me.

Control Is an Illusion

June 8, 2010

SO MUCH OF MY RECENT thinking about my life and my childless condition has focused on letting go. An essential step in the letting go process is realizing we have no control over any person, place, or thing. That is incredibly difficult for me. With all of the tragedies in my life, I have created a facade of control. If I do this, then that won't happen. If only it worked that way.

I just got back from the ICU where my friend of 25 years' father lay on a respirator after suffering a catastrophic stroke. He's young. She had just talked to him a couple of hours before. Now, it is very likely he will not recover. Obviously, if I could have stopped this from happening, I would have, but that is not my point here. Life is seemingly normal one minute, and literally minutes later, it's not.

A friend of mine told me today I have good coping skills and that is why I have managed to keep on going even though my life has been turned to shit more than once. I continue to wonder how I developed such coping skills, and if they are beneficial. In my present situation, they seem to be more of a hindrance than a help.

Following Samantha's murder, I pretty much lost my mind for a while. Once I collected myself (well, mostly), I got a job at the local convenience store. I worked midnight shift and saw the same people night after night buying beer and cigarettes. One person in particular, Ralph, would come to my window every single night at 1 a.m. and buy a case of beer and a pack of Marlboros. He always looked tired and a little sad.

One night around midnight as I cleaned the butter from the sides of the popcorn machine, I saw Ralph stroll up to the window, an hour early. This time he ordered two cases of beer. Evidently, Ralph was in for a night of extra heavy drinking. I decided that night I did not want to become like Ralph. I decided to go back to high school (I dropped out in March of my senior year). I did just that.

What was is it that made me go back to high school? What made me think that I could have a better life?

My motivation was simple: I promised myself I would never allow a man to control my life or my children's lives. I would never be trapped in a bad relationship. And the only way out of that lot in life seemed to be an education. So back to high school I went.

However, in my quest to not allow someone to control me, I not only tried to control myself but everyone and everything in my life. I would not be hurt again! My future children would never be hurt!

It doesn't work like that.

While I still agree that being economically independent is essential to my wellbeing, I have come to realize healthy interdependence with others is also essential. Rather than trying to control others to ensure my preferred outcome, I need to work with others to get the BEST outcome, which might not be the one I have imagined.

When I met my husband nearly 17 years ago, I was absolutely smitten. He walked through the door of the student union and I knew immediately I wanted "that one." However, he wasn't ready and now, I am sure I wasn't either. All these years later, we are together and in a much better place than we were then. Therefore, if I would have gotten my wish, we might never have made it.

Maybe the same is true with the baby situation. Things don't happen on my time table. In fact, some things never happen.

I am not the type of person to let things ride. I have trouble allowing the world to turn on its own. It scares me to go with the flow. I am usually a happy-go-lucky person with the small things in life...but economic security, romance, and having child are big areas in which I feel like I have to control.

I can't.

Acceptance is a requirement. I must accept I have done all I can do to bring a healthy baby home. I cannot change my reality.

Fulton Oursler has said, "Many of us crucify ourselves between two thieves—regret for the past and fear of the future." I have acknowledged my regrets and I must stop fearing a childless future.

On Sunday I did two very different, yet related things. I went to a barbecue at my in-laws and I took a canoe down a flooded creek. The barbecue at my in-laws was a going away party for my sister-in-law. At the barbecue, my nephew had his two little girls...four and two. Usually, it is painful for me to be around them. But I refuse to let it hurt me anymore. In fact, at some point I found myself pushing the oldest one on a swing. Normally, she is shy and reserved, but as she went higher and higher, she began talking. We had a good time together. And for the first time in a long time, I wasn't screaming inside because I don't have a child of my own.

Following the barbecue, my husband and I decided to take our canoe for its maiden voyage. The creek near our house was flooded, and it was the perfect time to go for a ride. I was worried about getting tossed out of the boat; canoes are notorious for flipping. But I went for that ride and loved every minute of it, even when we were tossed over a dam and the boat took on water. We didn't fall out. We just kept on floating along.

These two events taught me I can face my fears. I can spend time with children without drowning in grief and I can sail a boat on a flooded creek without drowning in its murky brown waters. I won't be crippled by fear of the unknown any longer. I do not know my life without children would be miserable. After all, it hasn't been. And I did not know if I would fall in the water. As my favorite band, Over the Rhine, sings:

> *Obsessions with self-preservation*
> *Faded when I threw my fear away*
> *It's not a thing you can imagine*
> *You either lose your fear*
> *Or spend your life with one foot in the grave*

I don't want to spend any more of my days with one foot leaning more towards death than life. Life is short, and as my friend discovered today, it is also fleeting. It can change in an instant, for good and ill. I can't stop that, but I can determine how I will live each day.

A Disease of the Imagination

June 12, 2010

NOW I HAVE turned the corner towards acceptance of childlessness, I have been pondering why acceptance is such an incredible challenge. One reason, I think, it is so difficult to deal with not having children is lack of imagination.

I have spent so much of my life imagining what it will be like when I have children. What kind of parent I would be. What kind of school I would send my children to. How I would establish and maintain rules. All of those are good mental exercises when preparing for an enormous job such as parenting. The problem is I created this fantasy future with such great detail that I have been having the worst time dismantling it. I find it even challenging to supplant it with another dream.

Therefore, I have realized I am suffering a deficit of imagination. I just don't have enough at this point in time to change the future I dreamed for myself, and perhaps that is the actual problem.

I am high on the goal-setting spectrum. I could never have achieved all I have achieved in my life without being able to set goals and reach them. After all, you don't just stumble onto a Ph.D. Nonetheless, all that obsessive goal work has led to a real lack in living each day to its fullest. Lately, I have been getting better at that, but it is still a struggle. I firmly believe if you don't have dreams then you can never get out of a bad situation.

So, I am at an impasse when it comes to having children. How do I let go of the future I imagined for myself and my imaginary child?

One way I am doing that is by recognizing the need I have around me. There are young people in my life who can use the skills I bring to the table; nieces and nephews who have good parents but who could use a bit more adult presence in their lives. I am also considering signing up for Big Brothers, Big Sisters. I really seem to have a knack with working with girls 13-16. They seem to relate to me and my sense of reality. If I can use that gift to help other people's children, then why not?

At one point during the throes of the fertility drug madness, I told my husband I would kill myself if I found out I could never have children. I have reconsidered that statement completely since then. It is ridiculous to think life would not be worth living without children when so much of my life is so very good.

One of the actions they encourage in Al-Alon is to make a gratitude list when you are feeling bad. I end this post with my gratitude list. Not that I am feeling bad, but because I am feeling especially grateful.

I am grateful for...
- good friends who stand next to me through troubled times
- a job I love going to even on bad days

- a beautiful home that is warm and welcoming to all who enter it
- a flourishing garden that continues to put food on my table
- two wonderful cats who keep me company night and day
- a caring husband who tries as hard as I do to keep our marriage going
- a car that gets me to work and back without fail
- a freelance career that helps pay the bills and keeps me busy over the summers
- a computer that makes my work easier

I must remember even though my dreams have changed, I have not. In my core I am still me, and I still have, as Over the Rhine sings, "a lust for life and an iron will." I really do believe if I can see it, then I can be it. Sometimes I just misinterpret what I see.

The Devil's in the Details

June 13, 2010

LATELY, I HAVE BEEN talking a good game. Working on acceptance and letting go. And I really have been trying my best. I knew it wouldn't be easy, so I expected some slips along the way. And, of course, I've had a couple.

My husband and I had an argument last night about my decision to stop actively trying to get pregnant. He said I did not talk about it with him. I said I tried several times, but he would walk away or change the subject or say, "Enough." And it seemed to me it didn't matter to him one way or the other. I know he said he wanted kids, but his lack of interest and participation in the fertility treatments seemed to suggest otherwise.

Evidently, I was wrong.

I asked him why he waited until now to say something. He answered with silence.

I certainly never meant to exclude him from this decision. I explained to him I would not try to prevent conception but I would no longer seek medical assistance in trying to get pregnant. I guess since the drugs and charting and testing and everything else was directly effecting me that it really is my decision. No one should make a person or even WANT to make a person go through that who doesn't wish to. I apologized to him for not considering his feelings in this, but I urged him not to try and change my mind because I really have had enough.

And then I woke up this morning to my period.

I guess as long as my period still hadn't started since the surgery it was easy for me to ignore the entire TTC debacle. Nothing can be done — no tests run, no pills taken, nothing — until the beginning of the menstrual cycle, and it arrived today and shook my world up, but only a bit.

I tried to talk to him this morning about the TTC decision, but he jumped up from the table and said he had to go clean the garage. Rather than sulking about it, I took it as a good moment. If we don't talk about it, then there is no way I will feel the slightest urge to pick up the phone and ask for fertility meds. And yet now I wonder if I should go through with getting that repeat HSG (the dye test needed to prove that my right tube is indeed open as expected).

Part of me dreads the thought of having that test done again. It will be the fourth time!

Another part of me thinks that I MUST do it to prove to myself that the tube is indeed open.

And yet another part of me is scared to death to find out that it is blocked, which would leave no possibility of spontaneous pregnancy.

(There are more parts of me than I thought!)

So now I am confused. This acceptance thing is difficult! As much as I would welcome a child into my life, the idea of continuing this obsessive quest is repugnant to me. I used to fear the day when I would have to stop trying, and now I welcome it with open arms.

My brother and his pregnant girlfriend visited me today. It was a little bit painful, especially when my brother asked me about my journey to get pregnant.

"Are there any new developments? Maybe it is time to think about adoption."

I didn't tell him that I had stopped trying. It would be too difficult and too painful to explain. I simply said, "No. Nothing new."

And then he pointed to his girlfriend's shirt, which read, "I'm not fat. I am pregnant." I laughed, but it hurt a little, just a little.

Later, while we were talking on my deck, the baby kicked and she said, "The baby must like you because every time you talk, it moves." And that hurt, a lot. I remembered the last time I felt a child move inside me, and I took a long, slow, deep breath. But before the pain gave way to terrible sadness, I looked over at my nephew, 15, and I thought about how much I love him and how happy I am to have him in my life and to be spending an evening with him, and the pain vanished. He started laughing about something his Dad said, and my heart filled with joy to see his face light up with happiness.

I haven't healed from this grief, but I am finding ways to heal. I am reaching towards joy and turning my back on sorrow. After all, the life my brother's girlfriend is carrying is one that I will be able to share. I will hold that child one day and watch him or her grow up. There is no need for me to be envious or to hurt because I am not pregnant and because I do not have living children of my own. After all, I have a wonderful nephew who is willing to spend a stunning summer evening with his aunt doing nothing but talking and drinking iced tea. I am truly blessed to have all that I have in this life. I just need only to receive those gifts.

Like Over the Rhine sings, "There's nothing harder than learning how to receive." Until now, I wasn't quite sure what they meant, but I do know I must not focus on the empty chair (or in my case, the empty bedroom) and rather at the crowded sofa that is overflowing with more happiness than I can ever deplete.

This Me, That Me

June 16, 2010

I ALMOST MADE THE CALL. Several times today, I had the phone in my hand ready to make the appointment for the HSG. Yet, I didn't. The thought of it fills me with such dread that I can't even think about getting in the car and driving to the hospital, let alone having the procedure done and then, getting the results.

In one way, I guess it would be better to get the test done. If the right tube is blocked, then I will know all bets are off and I can stop being anxious about it all. Maybe tomorrow.

I have been thinking about all of the women who would jump at the chance to have IVF, even if they had to wait a year. I used to be one of those women. There was a time when the very thought of IVF seemed so farfetched that I never bothered to do research on it. That me would be shocked that this me would ever walk away from it. And yet here I am.

There was a certain amount of comfort in the fact I knew then that IVF was off the table forever. It was never a possibility. It forced me to consider an end point for TTC. After Clomid or some other ovulation-inducing drug, then that was it. The end of the line. My ex-h and I agreed to walk away after that.

In fact, I was ready to stop trying altogether until my house burned down in 2004.

My seven cats died in that fire, and although I was close to all of them, I was closest to Wladek. He and his sister, Mila, and their brother, Mishka, were found behind Ellis Hall at Ohio University on the Monday after Mother's Day in 2003. They were three hours old when I bundled them up in my sweatshirt and took them home. My ex-h and I became their surrogate parents. We fed them with a syringe every two hours, bathed them, and helped them pee. We warmed their bed with a heating pad and introduced them to our older cats. We were told by our vet their chance of survival was less than 20%. Having lost our son Nicholas in 2001, the idea of losing these three newborns was unfathomable. Sadly, we lost Mishka when he was three weeks old. But Wladek and Mila went on to become enormous black cats. I fell hopelessly in love with Wladek.

Wlad followed me around like I was his mother. He slept under my shirt or on my shoulder. He would get into bed every single morning when my alarm went off and lay his head on my head and curl his tail around my neck. To say that I was attached to him is too mild of a word. I recall very fondly reciting Elizabeth Barrett Browning's poem to him as he sat high up on the banister:

> *How do I love thee? Let me count the ways.*
> *I love thee to the depth and breadth and height*
> *My soul can reach, when feeling out of sight*
> *For the ends of Being and ideal Grace.*

Then, the house burned down, and he died inside. What was left of my heart washed away in a gully of tears. I still miss him. I miss his voice. His face. His constant, loving presence. Although I went on to adopt two wonderful cats, the place that Wlad filled in my heart remains empty.

When Wlad was alive, I was willing to accept not having children. I could have coped then. He needed me. I needed him. He let me be his Mama, and I enjoyed every second of it. People who have never had a special relationship with an animal may not understand how my relationship with Wlad could be so fulfilling, but it was, and I could have lived the rest of his days mostly content without children.

Following my divorce in 2007, I began dating my college sweetheart (my husband), and he told me he wanted children. And so began the obsession anew.

I am trying to get back to that point of contentment. Although my marriage was in deep trouble by the time the house burned down, my feelings towards childlessness were those of peace and a tad bit of longing. Perhaps it was because my marriage was in trouble, but I really believe it was because my relationship with Wlad was so fulfilling.

As I move closer towards letting go, I search for fulfillment elsewhere in my life. If it is true a negative behavior (TTC obsession) must be replaced with positive behavior, then I need to find a positive focus for my attention. At this point, focusing on my overall health and on my relationships with the young people in my life seem to make the most sense. Both of these areas would be worthy of attention by this me AND that me.

Living in the Moment

June 21, 2010

AND SO I MADE that appointment for the HSG test. It is on Thursday, and I am going to go. I put it off, and I really thought I would skip it, but then my own curiosity got the better of me. I want to know if that tube is blocked. If it is, then there will never be a time when I think I am pregnant and obsess over the symptoms because if it is blocked, there is no way I can get pregnant without the help of IVF. I have decided not to tell my husband about this procedure. I am just going to go and get it done.

On the upside, I am getting better at living in the moment. In the past week I have had chance to spend quite a bit of time with one of my nieces and one of my nephews, and the entire time we were together, I tried to live in the moment and enjoy every second.

I am starting to appreciate more the many blessings I have in my life, and not be weighed down by what I don't have. All in all, I have a pretty great life, and I know I must embrace it as it is. Never before in my life have I had so much love, friendship, and economic wellbeing. It would be much more than just a shame to let this time of my life pass me by without appreciating it fully.

In this great article in *Psychology Today*, the author talks about the art of now, living in the moment. One of the strongest messages is "you are not your thoughts." That is incredibly hard for me to accept, but I am getting there, one step at a time.

Mindfulness certainly seems like a blessing so far. I wonder if there was ever a time beyond the very early years of my life I have ever been able to or was willing to try to live in the now? I guess after Samantha was murdered I attempted to do so because ruminating about the past was horrifying. Other than that, I have been obsessed with the future and the past. And you see where that got me...

Wisdom! Be Attentive!

June 23, 2010

My ex-husband is Ukrainian Catholic, and I loved to go to mass with him. There was something about the combination of incense, Cyrillic, and chanting that spoke to me. Unlike the Catholic masses I had attended, the Ukrainian Catholic masses seemed sensual and embodied.

One of my favorite parts of the mass was when the priest would walk around with an enormous Bible and shout "Wisdom! Be Attentive!" It was as if he was saying, "Good stuff, coming through. You better listen or you'll miss it." And I listened!

Wisdom! Be Attentive!

Sometimes I don't listen when wisdom is present and that is something I am trying to change. Two incidents this past week made me stand up and take notice.

One afternoon, I was in the grocery store looking for cheese for the tacos I was making for dinner that night. As I strolled down the dairy aisle, I saw two elderly people in motorized carts talking, and I admired one of the men's hats. It was a suede cowboy hat decorated with a ring of Christmas goodies: bows, holly, berries, bears. Even though it was the official first day of summer, there was something about all that holiday swag that made me smile.

As I walked by, he smiled and said hello. I smiled back and told him I admired his hat. He said he admired my headscarf, which has become my constant summer adornment. We started chatting, and he relayed to me his life wisdom. He was about to "turn 79 on August 30," so he had quite a lot to say. Although I could have walked away at any time, I thought maybe I could learn something from him, and sure enough, I did.

He told me he could tell by the way I held myself I am a confident and caring person. He reminded me that looks, fake or real, fade and all we have left, especially at his age, are our thoughts and memories. He also said if a person really believes in something, then it can come true. He is obviously not a man of means, but he seemed content with how his life turned out. As I walked away he pelted me with platitudes:

"Treat others how you wish to be treated."

"Don't sweat the small stuff."

"A penny saved is a penny earned."

And, of course, all of his talk about dreams and goals started me back on the "wishing for a baby track," which as you know, I have been trying quite hard to jump from. I left there thinking, "Maybe... if only I ... you know I could ..." but by the time I pulled into my driveway, I had found my resolve and was once again extolling the benefits of not having children.

Then, I had another encounter.

I went swimming at a lake yesterday with a friend from my college days. It was wonderful! Fresh, clean water with a sand bottom. I could have stayed there for days. Following our swim, I met my friend's godfather and owner of the lake and campgrounds. Within minutes it was clear I needed to be attentive.

Like me, he had discovered that positive thinking and being open to the universe are powerful ways of living. It is not about acquisition but about finding peace and enjoying life in a way that had seemed illusive previously. As he explained his philosophy of life to me, I couldn't help but jump in with all I had recently read and pondered. We had a lot in common, but I could tell he had been at this way of thinking for far longer than I had been, so I listened carefully.

He asked many questions, and I gladly gave him the answers. He assured me if I truly believed something would come true, then it would. He cited many examples from his own life where just that had happened. He asked me what I wanted. I told him that I had wanted to have children.

He said, "You still do."

He then said to achieve that goal I needed to articulate the want (check), pray about it (check), and let it go (um, ...).

I asked him why letting go was so hard.

He said, "Because it is."

As we talked I felt like I was standing before the Delphic oracle or maybe chatting with Aristotle. In any case, he offered me much more wisdom, and I am pondering it. His main message was not new, "See it. Believe it. Be it."

And now I am in the middle of a quandary: Go back to hoping and believing that I will one day have a child or continue on my path of letting go of that dream. Is it possible that they are the same thing? That maybe I have been looking at this situation all wrong. That instead of letting go of the dream itself, I need to let go of the belief that I can force it to happen by sheer will?

In any case, I feel irritated again. Partly because I am in fear of sliding back into my obsessive state, which was ruining my quality of life, and partly because I feel angry and resentful towards my husband because I truly believe he promised me something (IVF) and did not deliver. I could do it on my own economically, but it would cause a serious rift between us. I am fighting against feeling helpless because that is not true at all. But powerless might be an okay state because that is the true source of letting go.

I have my HSG appointment tomorrow. I will find out the initial results during the test. At this point, I dread the answer, but I am going to walk in and face the music. I have not told my husband about it. Sometimes things are easier to handle alone.

And the Results Are In

June 24, 2010

THE HSG IS OVER. It was far less painful than it has been in the past, so I am relieved. However, the fight that followed took some of the joy out of the positive results.

The procedure went very quickly, and my doctor announced the right tube is open and I can conceive naturally. He recommended I make an appointment to see him and he thinks we have many more options than just IVF and what we have been doing. I was buoyed by the news and left the hospital far happier and less anxious than when I walked in.

I waited for about an hour before I called my husband. I wanted to enjoy the good news for a while without the cloud of darkness that I figured he would hang over it. He did not answer my call, and I breathed a sigh of relief. I did a little shopping for the beach trip we are going on this weekend, and enjoyed what remained of my afternoon. When he finally called me back, I could hear in his voice that he was angry and upset. I braced myself all the way home for what would most likely be a fight.

Sure enough, our conversation about the results of the procedure disintegrated into an argument about the fertility process that ended with him saying, "You don't think I am good enough for you." I asked for him to be more supportive. Although I would never have put it the way he interpreted it, I guess he is right. Being a quarter of the way involved is not good enough.

In my readings as of late, one thing I have learned is that a lot of anger comes from not having needs met. One way to overcome that type of anger is to ask that your needs be met. I asked him for the following:

1. To come to the follow-up meeting with me in July. At this meeting, my doctor will go over options with me. If he is there, then he can learn about those options and we can make a decision together.
2. To be supportive of me when I am undergoing stress, including when I am approaching a major hormonal shift from pills or just the normal changes in my cycle.
3. To not get angry when I let him know I am in my fertile period and need to have sex.

I don't think these needs are unrealistic. He does. He accused me of making him dance like a marionette. He says I am controlling.

I said, "If you want to have a child, then you have to be part of this. I cannot and will not do it alone."

He blew up again.

I know this is stressful for him, but we are not going be less stressed out if we fight and continue not working together. I explained if things go like they did over the seven months I was taking fertility drugs I was not going to do it again. He said nothing.

We are now sitting in silence. He is watching a movie. I am blogging. We are supposed to be headed to the beach in the morning. I am worried about the trip. I just want to enjoy the ocean, but I feel like it will be harder than ever to relax and let go. However, I am sure once I see that forever horizon stretching out before me I will be unable to hold my breath any longer.

Catch a Wave and You're Sittin' on Top of the World

June 29, 2010

I WENT ON A BIT of a hiatus to take a beach vacation. We had talked about going for a month or two, but we weren't really sure when we were going. A couple of hours after I posted my last entry, we loaded up the car and took off with no reservations, and no concrete plans. It turned out to be one of the best things we could have done.

Following our enormous fight on Thursday evening, we both realized we need to just go and let go. We did just that and did not quarrel from the moment we shut the trunk and headed east. We drove all night and landed on the Atlantic coast at Ocean City at 6 a.m. Friday morning. The ocean was too hard to resist, and we scrambled to the beach, soaking our clothes and shoes as we waded deep into the salty water.

We spent hours on the beach and forgot about our troubles. Trying to conceive was on my mind, but only briefly and only because I was gearing up to ovulate. Otherwise, I did my best to live in the moment, to enjoy every second of the cool, blue water and my husband's company. It was the honeymoon we never had. We were so busy when we got married with buying the house, moving, and school starting we did not have chance to do more than have a nice dinner at Oglebay Park, but our weekend on the beach was better than any honeymoon we could have planned.

We took a moonlit walk on a deserted part of the beach. The moon was full and the ocean was calm. We held hands and talked softly to each other, unwilling to even consider the rarity of such a moment. We were living for the now not for tomorrow, next week, or last year.

But the most specific lesson to be learned from our trip was learned in the water.

I had been to the beach before, but back then (about nine years ago) I was so worried about how I looked in a bathing suit I wouldn't go in the water. I wore a cover up and concealed as much of myself as I could. Thankfully, I have lost most of that self-consciousness and I was stripped down to my swimsuit in minutes.

Although I swim daily in my sister-in-law's pool (and sometimes at the Y), the ocean is still overwhelming. Nothing else on Earth makes me feel as humble as the ocean. It is so much bigger and more powerful than me. It is a clear representation of my Higher Power.

This force is made even more apparent when you try to swim in the ocean. Just getting off the shore and into the water takes incredible effort as each wave batters swimmers with its white frothy force. I went down over and over again that first day. I tried diving head first into each wave and ended up being tossed to the ocean floor and dragged across the gravely sand.

For hours I kept trying to find a rhythm. The kids next to me made it seem so easy. My husband tried to help. But for some reason all I earned for my effort was matted hair and scraped knees. I was enjoying myself, but in an exhaustive way. In fact, the harder I tried, the harder I fell.

After recovering overnight, I headed back out into the water, determined to find a way to ride the waves and not let them pummel me for hours.

At first I approached entry the same way I had the day before: I eased in and braced myself, thinking I could somehow withstand its cruel, but awesome strength. Once again, I was thrown to the shore, gasping for air and trying with little success to stand back up before the next wave hit. I struggled to my feet and stomped back to my beach blanket in disgust. I was disappointed in myself.

After brooding for a bit, I collected myself and gave it another shot. This time I would let go. I pushed my way to the flat, soft sand and surrendered. Instead of fighting the next wave as it came in, I relaxed and it lifted me up and back to the shore. I did not get thrashed. Instead, I glided on the crest of the wave and landed gently on the ocean floor. I spent the rest of the day and all of the next giggling and dancing in the surf. Yes, I got pounded a few more times, but I recovered quickly and eventually began to look forward to the biggest waves.

At one point I told my husband for the first time I understood the immense power in letting go. I have been trying to let go of the obsession of having children, but the trying was preventing it from happening. I learned as I struggled to outlast the ocean when something is beyond my control the best way to survive it (and even enjoy it!) is to surrender to it.

Several entries ago, I quoted from Toni Morrison's fabulous novel, *Song of Solomon:* "If you surrender to the air, then you can ride it." The same is true of the ocean. I surrendered, and I rode wave after wave. Although I never knew quite where I would end up after each wave subsided, I did know I would eventually find my way back to shore. I have never felt so peaceful. I found true contentment. Not once while I was being buoyed by the rolling waves did I think about what I was lacking in life. I thought only about the next wave and Jim's strong arms he would occasionally slip around my waist to pull me to him so that we could ride a wave together. We discovered that we were stronger together as one.

Applying what I learned to my TTC struggle is challenging but more than worth the effort. To not actively try to get pregnant by minding my cycles and even taking fertility drugs or undergoing some other kind of treatment is risky. I am not getting any younger.

However, only half living my life because I am consumed with having a child is just as risky. What might I miss (and have missed) by doing so? I might never have children. I understand that. But I am not going to dwell on it. Instead, I am going to surrender to life. I will work on what I can accomplish and let the rest of it go. Instead of charging at it without regard for its power and getting thrown to the punishing sand, I will relax and keep my eye on the next wave that comes rolling in, not to try to fight it off, but to see where it takes me.

July 2010

Inside My Hula Hoop

July 1, 2010 at 10:01 pm

ONE OF AL ANON'S slogans focuses on minding what is inside your hula hoop. In other words, you should only be concerned with what is your business and not anyone else's. Worrying about what goes on in other people's lives will only make your life miserable. After all, no one can change anyone else. We can only change ourselves. However...

Yesterday I learned that someone I know who is pregnant continues to smoke pot daily. Although I could care less what adults do in their free time, I was immediately concerned by this news. I hold my breath going through tunnels (the poisonous gasses can cause birth defects in the first trimester), never eat deli meats or cheeses (the risk of salmonella exposure is too high), and avoid alcoholic when I THINK I could be pregnant. I cannot imagine using a drug when I KNOW that I have a child growing inside of me.

Obviously, I am having trouble minding only what's inside my hula hoop.

I did a little bit of research about marijuana use in pregnancy. The results are mixed. Some studies have found that it has limited impact on developing fetuses, while others show that it can cause severe birth defects. The majority of studies, however, show that regular use of pot during pregnancy causes children to develop ADHD later in life. The most serious side effects are associated with daily use, including low birth weight, pre-term delivery, and nervous system disorders.

People who have tried to talk to her about it are given the same response: "My doctor says it's okay and better than cigarettes." I wonder...

I am left to ponder this situation. I know that her actions are endangering her unborn child's development, but I also know that if I say anything that my words will either go unheeded or aggravate the situation. I know I cannot make her stop. It is just so hard to do nothing.

I must learn, though, that there are things I really have no control over. And in many ways that is good. If I had control over everything, then I would go insane trying to make the world a better place—according to me. I must accept that my worldview is not the ONLY one. Also, it is not necessarily right or wrong. The same is true of the views of others.

As I look towards the weekend of Independence that approaches, I cannot help but think about freedom. Where does my personal freedom begin and where does it end? And the freedom of others? If we must "live and let live," where is the line drawn? If making a statement or taking action will not affect change, then is their any point to doing either? If stepping outside of my hula hoop will not help me or anyone else, shouldn't I just stay inside it and hope for the best?

The Universe Will Provide (But You Gotta Help)

July 5, 2010 at 7:07 pm

FOLLOWING BEING LEFT in the middle of nowhere on Friday, we tried to reconcile but only ended up fighting more, especially in couple's counseling the next morning. As we searched for a way to get past our troubles, I opened my heart and mind, and our healing took the form of a camping trip to the mountains.

It is difficult to forgive your partner when he or she hurts you. At times it is so difficult for me that I would rather call it quits than try to work through the anguish that forgiveness sometimes requires. I kept waiting for him to say or do something to make the pain of his words go away when I really needed to look inside myself.

He apologized, and I did not accept. It seemed feeble and insincere. He then turned it all back on me, accusing me of leaving him. (It made no sense, so it was both outrageous and hilarious. After all, he drove away.) At one point, he said, "I am sorry that I left you there. I really thought you wanted me to go so that you could be with your friends. I am not perfect, but I am trying so hard. I am trying harder than any other time in my life."

His words made me remember that I am not perfect either. I say things that I shouldn't and do things that are hurtful to him, too.

Despite that knowledge, I was unable to move beyond the moment, that feeling of being abandoned and then being treated like I was not worthy of his care. The promise of an impromptu trip to the mountains of West Virginia helped me reach towards peace.

We loaded the car quickly, kissed the cats goodbye, and drove off late in the evening towards the middle of the state. We had both been there enough to know the lay of the land, but we had no campsite reservation and it was Fourth of July weekend. We both felt that all would be well when we got there, wherever "there" specifically meant.

We found our site at 11:05 pm, after driving through two fireworks displays and miles of dark mountain roads. It was a perfect site with a fire pit, plenty of firewood, and flat ground for our tent. Our headlights illuminated the rhododendrons and pine trees that would serve as a backdrop for our stay.

We were so cold that night. It was 46 degrees, and we came ill prepared. I tried toughing it out in the tent, but the cold ground beneath me and the cold air pressing against the tent walls drove me to the car's heated seats and heater. Jim slept in the tent, swaddled in all of the blankets, coats, and towels that we could find in the car.

Throughout our trip and on into the cold night, we worked together. First to find the free camping zone in the Monongahela National Forrest and then to set up camp. We did not fight. Instead, we laughed together at our willingness to take a chance on finding a good campsite and then again at building a good fire.

We spent our Fourth hiking to all of our favorite spots: Table Rock, Blackwater Falls, Lindy Point. On one of our many hikes, we ran across a couple biking from the Falls to the main road. We chatted with them, and they chuckled at our brazeness to take a sedan down a mountain road that four-wheel drive jeeps would be lucky to navigate. They went on their way, and we turned our car around, fearing getting hung up or worse! Exhausted, we decided to stock up on supplies and spend one more night in our little mountain nook.

To make our night warmer, Jim inflated our queen-sized air bed using a car adapter and an air pump. At one point, I told him that it would probably run the battery down. He assured me that it would not draw that much power. We ended our evening snuggled in bed after an evening of guitar playing and singing around our campfire.

In the morning we discovered that the battery had died. The familiar click, click, click meant a hike out of the forest in search of a helping hand.

As we strapped on our hiking shoes, Jim apologized for the situation that he felt he got us into. I told him not to worry, that if we opened our minds and hearts to the universe, help would come.

Within 15 minutes of our hike, we spotted a man jogging with his dog. As he got closer, we realized that he was the man we had crossed paths with the morning before as he and his wife biked along the road. He recognized us immediately and agreed to give us a jump. In less than 20 minutes we were on our way home. Thank yous and well wishes exchanged. During our hike, I never stopped believing that our helper would arrive quickly. I didn't even have time to have doubts.

I realized from this weekend, especially from this last part, that being kind to others pays off in big dividends and that the universe will provide for everyone, it just might not be when and how we wish things to be. I also learned, again, that Jim and I are never stronger or closer than when we are in dire straits, like when we were holding hands while catching enormous waves at the ocean last weekend.

Of course, this brings me back to my biggest wish: having children. Will it ever happen? When? In what form?

All I can do is open my heart and mind open to the possibility—and keep them open. I won't sit around and wait for whatever the universe has in store for me, but I will hike the path of life believing that the resolution is just around the bend (or across the mountain).

Playing with Fire

July 7, 2010 at 9:24 pm

AT SOME POINT, I am going to have to face it. I haven't opened the plastic tubs since I put the photo albums in there shortly after they were rescued from the ruins of the house. Having opened the other, very few, boxes of items "saved" from the house fire, I know that as soon as I lift the lids, I will be greeted by the acrid smell of smoke and ash. Yet if I am going to start scrapbooking (and in some ways, living) again, I am going to have to take off those lids.

It is ironic that I would be edging towards this moment today.

Soon after I had made up my mind to take the two purple, Rubbermaid tubs out of my office storage area, Jim called to say that his truck was on fire. He was stranded in the mountains of Maryland for nearly four hours as the fire was put out and re-ignited on its own several times. Thankfully, fellow trucks stopped to lend him a hand, but the heat of the day and the waiting has exhausted his mind and body. Although the truck is inoperable and may never run again, business went on, and he is pulling his load with a replacement cab to its destination.

However, fires aren't always so innocuous.

As I have mentioned here, my house burned down in 2004 just five days before Christmas. I lost everything, including my six beloved cats. In addition, I lost 22 years of writing, my wedding dress, and my children's blankets and other mementos. Although I lost an album of childhood family photos, my high school yearbook, and my college scrapbook, the fire chief was able to save several albums of photos, including my wedding album and my son's pictures. When he placed the charred books in my arms, I was stunned that they were in such good shape. While they certainly did not look like they did they day I put them together, I felt that I could work with the plastic coated pages and re-make them or at least save the pictures.

Nearly six years later, they remain in the boxes that I stored them in.

I have tried lifting the lids several times, but the thought of the stench of that December night wafting out at me repels me. But I know that if I am ever going to pull the pieces of my life back together again, I must do this. I must look through those pages and see what I can save.

One night during our recent camping trip Jim watched as I burned my marshmallows to a cinder. I love them that way! He said, "I think you just like to play with fire." I had never thought about that before. One thing I cannot live without during the summer is a good campfire, but in the summers following the house fire, I could not stand the smell of wood burning. I guess I have moved past that now, but I still live in fear of another house fire. More cats dying in a suffocating blaze. Losing it all all over again.

Two weeks ago, I heard the siren and watched as a fire truck screamed down my street (I was driving the other direction). I whipped my car around and chased the truck, praying that it would not stop in front of my house. It slowed as it approached the corner of my block, and I nearly threw up with fear, knowing that it was my house. My cats. My life. Again.

Thankfully, it sped by and headed up the hill. I quietly prayed for the people at the truck's destination, but nearly fell while jumping out of my car and rushing in the front door. Although I know that to some extent such anxiety is to be expected–after all, I found out my other house was on fire by seeing the smoke on my way across town–I also know that I have to put this behind me.

In many ways I have moved on. I adopted other cats, though not as replacements. My kitties could never be replaced. I no longer turn off the furnace when I go away for more than a few hours in the winter. I don't have nightmares anymore. And yet there is still a struggle within me to move forward and free myself of the mental torture that baseless fear has over me. I have done it before. For example, I was able to get over the fear of dying during pregnancy or childbirth, even though both have been close calls for me in the past.

So tomorrow when I am alone, I will take off those lids (wearing gloves and a face mask, of course) and see what I can save and what must be discarded. They are pictures of my past and will no doubt resurrect bittersweet memories. In fact, images of my second marriage exist only in those boxes. I can face the past. It is the only way to welcome the future.

Opening Pandora's Boxes

July 8, 2010 at 5:23 pm

OKAY, SO THEY ARE NOT really boxes, but plastic tubs, but still. I wasn't quite sure what I would find when I lifted those lids. Would the pictures be charred beyond recognition? Would the albums be too moldy to save? Would the plastic page covers be adhered to the images? Latex gloves and face mask donned, I took off the first lid.

I took the tubs out one at a time. The smell of smoke, ash and melted plastic remained but was nowhere near as strong as it was when last I lifted those lids. Since you aren't here, I thought I would take some pictures so I wouldn't be so alone on my journey.

I opened the first purple tub and saw what I knew to be enclosed therein. Several photo albums with spines burned, melted, and falling apart. As I pulled each one out, I marveled at the exterior damage.

I was surprised when I opened each book to find that many of the pictures, when removed from their plastic sleeves, were in excellent condition.

In fact, I should be able to remove many of the pages in each album to clean albums without doing much repair.

A double-page spread of my 30th birthday pictures. The corners of each page were licked with smoke, but otherwise, the photos suffered no fire or water damage.

Of course, not everything was saved. I found a couple of stacks of photos fused together by what I think was water. There is no way to separate them and save the images.

As I continued to dig through the first box, I found photos! Hundreds and hundreds of photos with their negatives, including copies of most of the ones that had been adhered to each other. I suddenly remembered finding them after the fire tucked safely in fire safe photo boxes. In fact, the ones in the boxes were in better shape than the ones in the albums. What a relief!

It turned out that opening the boxes wasn't the horrendous experience that I had anticipated. There were far more pictures in much better shape than I had remembered. I think I must have gone through them at some point before I stored them, but I have no memory of doing so.

I opened tub two with gusto, expecting to find other forgotten treasures, and I did! My college scrapbook, which I thought had been lost to the blaze, sat on top, along with scrapbooking supplies and more boxes of photos in perfect condition. I eager dug through the mess, but stopped immediately when I found a box in an oversized plastic bag.

I read his name, which was scrawled in my cursive script: Nicholas. Inside the box were items associated with my son. I did not remember that any of his things had been recovered from the house. Unlike the photo albums and boxes, his belongings were in a box in my bedroom closet, which was severely damaged by water and smoke. Evidently, the firemen had saved something of his.

At first I couldn't muster the courage to open the box. I walked into the kitchen and poured myself some iced tea. Then, I fed the cats. After that, I watered the flowers, turned on the TV, and checked my email. Slowly, I went back into the dining room and stared down into the tub at the bottom of the box. With shaking hands, I hauled it up, surprised to hear something rolling around inside.

I took the box out of the plastic bag and sat it on the table. I stared at it for quite some time and warily inched towards it, as though a poisonous snake lurked inside waiting to attack when I opened the lid.

I took a deep breath and revealed the contents.

I immediately began to cry. Inside the box, I found many of Nicholas' things: his frog that played "You are My Sunshine" as it hung by his bassinet, the candle from his memorial service, the face masks we used the last moment we saw him, his blanket (sadly, it has smoke damage), and perhaps most precious of all, the little bunny his Dad bought him. It sat next to his head under the cellophane wrap that kept his tiny body warm the short week that he lived.

As I held each item in my hand, I cried, reliving that bittersweet time of my life when I had my son in my arms and then lost him. I took the bunny out of its plastic case, and smelled it, trying to find the faintest hint of my boy, of the life that once lived inside of me. I wept for a long, long time both for the loss of my son and for joy at having found these wonderful things that connected me to him.

I pulled the chord on his green frog and listened to the tune that will always remind me of him and held his bunny in my arms. They were nearly the same size. We called Nicholas "Our Little Bunny," and this small, stuffed animal is a representation of him.

I knew there were pictures of Nicholas in the box, but I had no idea these items were anywhere, much less in a box next to my desk. I am not sure yet what I will do with them. I could put them in a memory box and display them, but doing doesn't seem right. I have photos of him and his sister in my living room, and they seem to be enough. I am sure that I will find a way to preserve them. I am just glad that they are safe and sound and within arm's reach.

As for all of the other photos, I am not sure. I started this purple tub quest because I had amassed so many photos from this summer that I wanted to start scrapbooking again. I have more than enough supplies, but I had turned away from scrapbooking after the fire and had never picked it up again. I enjoy it, but the weight of the recovered photos always held me back. In some ways, I felt that I could not create new scrapbooks while these other photos languished in boxes.

For now, I plan on storing them in clean albums and photo boxes. Whether I will build albums out of them in the future remains to be seen. I can imagine pulling out pictures of the cats and putting them into scrapbooks, but what about photos of me and my ex? How about our wedding album?

In some ways, it would have been easier if all of these things had been destroyed. If they were, then it would be easier to move on, to begin my life with Jim on a clean slate. But in reality, no one can never do that. Even if these artifacts had been lost forever, I still lived those days, months, and years. Even if, as I have found here, my memory, even my recent memory, is faulty, I still have impressions of that time. In addition, I am not at all ashamed of those years. In fact, much of my life with Nick was happy. We struggled financially, but we were good friends who were gifted with a little boy. Even though he lived only a week, we shared in that life together.

I know that finding Nicholas' things will help me along my TTC road. Healing comes in many forms and being reunited with my son's toys and blankets is part of that healing process. I must not have been ready to deal with them before now or else I would have remembered that they were saved and that I had kept them.

My excavating today was painful, joyful, and hopeful. At each turn I reminded myself of how lucky I am to have these remains. I have never been obsessed with acquiring objects. My life has focused on learning, building relationships with others, and self-improvement, but these artifacts serve as a link to my past and remind me once again that the universe has far more in store for me than I can even guess. I am eager to find out what is around the bend. Today I discovered another box marked "fire" in the basement. I think I just might have the courage to explore its contents after dinner.

The Vicious Cycle of Prayer

July 11, 2010 at 9:49 pm

I HAVE BEEN TRYING to figure out how prayer works since I was a child. I have turned to the Catholics, the Protestants, the pagans, and just about anyone I think might have an idea about the function and process of prayer, and I keep coming back to the same answer: prayer is a vicious cycle.

Let me explain my conundrum. Perhaps those of you who are wiser than me will be able to help.

If someone I love is dying, and I ask God (the universe, what/whoever) to not let that person die and that person does die, then does that mean that my prayer was for nothing? That I was unworthy of having my prayer answered? Why do some people live and other people die, even when they are prayed for my the same people with equal amounts of intensity?

Some people have said that it is not up to us to decide what is best in our lives and to ask for something specific, from as small as hitting a home run in the championship Little League game to being able to perform a successful open heart surgery, because only God (the universe, etc.) knows what is best for us.

So, what are we supposed to be prayer about?

The other night at an Al-Anon meeting, a member said, "I always pray that God's will be done." Well, won't it even if you don't pray for it?

And where does all of this leave wishing? (Remember all that wishing I was doing when I started this blog.) Do I wish for something I want or for something for someone else? Well, what is that is not part of the divine plan? What about believing, really believing? I have come to believe that I do not know what is best for me in all situations, partly because I only have limited knowledge:

what has happened before and what is happening right at that moment. Future events can alter if something wished for was granted is actually good or not.

For example, I have been wishing for a child. What if that child would become another Jeffrey Dahmer or Hitler? Of course, I cannot read the future...

so then maybe I should pray for something to happen or not to happen?!?

I know that I have benefited by the power of prayer and positive thinking. After all, it is far easier to go into or recover from a bad situation with a quieted mind than an anxious one. And although prayers did not save my son, they sure helped me feel stronger. I believe that I was able to get through that long, dark nightmare through that energy.

Perhaps that is the true power and purpose of prayer. A change of mindset, a calming of thought and heart, so that the next blow will be softened by the strength of being.

Thank You for Reading

July 13, 2010 at 1:29 am

I WANT TO TAKE the time to pause in my life reflections to thank you for reading along. I know that it takes time out of your day, but I cannot thank you enough for reading and for writing to me–here and in private–to let me know that you are sharing my introspections.

As I am sure all of you are aware enough to realize that what I post here are MY feelings and MY concerns. I try to understand others– sometimes desperately–but often fall short of getting past their own posturing and protective barriers. Most of us use those from time to time when we are frightened. Nonetheless, I think to be fully human our main concern is to understand ourselves. After all, we can control only ourselves. We cannot control others. I can control how I react to the words and deeds of others, but I surely cannot control what they say or do. At the same time, I am responsible only for myself, no one else. (And neither are you.)

One of my main goals recently has been to work on finding peace among chaos. This infertility journey has been difficult to traverse. Given that it has been going on for so long, at times I feel that the weight of it will crush me. Add in the mix the challenges of a new marriage, and it is a recipe for disaster. But that is why I write, and why I write as honestly as I can. I try to see myself for who I am, and I try to represent what I am going through with as much clarity as possible, but surely any intelligent reader should be able to see the pitfalls in writing about one's life. Unfortunately, other actors in that narrative do not always get their fair hearing, but given that this blog is about ME and MY feelings, I think that is just fine.

Many of you have written that you are thankful that I share my highs and lows because you can see yourself going through the same challenges. Some of you have said that I give you hope. I am glad to do it and glad to know that you are walking along on this journey with me. Those of you who are reading quietly, keep on doing so. I know you are out there, and you give me strength.

Thankfully, we are all grown ups here, and I think we all know that life is full of ups and downs. One day you think you might go crazy, and the next day you are riding on a wave at the ocean. I promise you, as I have in previous posts, that I will not censor my writing. I write from the heart and from the hip, and thank you for appreciating my honesty and for hanging in there with me through boring posts and posts written at the height of anger or tremendous joy.

Now, who is going to play me in the movie of my life? I always thought Nancy McKeon. You know, Jo from The Facts of Life. Until Hollywood comes knocking, I will keep on writing. I cannot tell you how much writing means to me and has meant to me throughout my life, and how much it means to me that you care about what I have to say.

Waiting for a Star to Fall

July 14, 2010

IT'S ONE O'CLOCK in the morning, and I cannot sleep. I figured I would write a little, to quiet my thoughts.

I just realized this morning my period is due in two days. No sign of the old girl just yet, but I am sure she will pop up just when I think the coast is clear. Intercourse timing was good this cycle. We were at the beach during ovulation, so we were relaxed and totally de-stressed. Unfortunately, I ovulated on my left side (the one without the tube), so the chances are pretty slim, but anything is possible.

This 2ww has been a breeze. I haven't been obsessing about symptoms, and I haven't even bought a pregnancy test. It is nice to not have TTC on my mind throughout the day. I have done far better than I thought I could. I guess my strategies are working.

I have an appointment with my reproductive endocrinologist in a couple of days. He is going to go over what he thinks are our next steps in the process should be. He said at the end of my HSG he thinks there is quite a bit we can do before turning to IVF, which gives me so much hope. I love my official doctor, but her partner (Dr. S) seems far more interested in my desired goals. My doctor insisted that IVF was the only solution, but Dr. S seems confident that truly will be a last resort.

It would be nice, though, to show up for my appointment with a positive pregnancy test, but even if that doesn't happen, I will be glad to hear what he has to say. The last time I saw him I was joking with him. I told him not to be alarmed when he performed the dye test and he can't find my left tube because he had taken it out about a month prior. He laughed and said he remembered it well. Life is funny, even when you are on a table four feet off the floor on your back with your legs in stirrups.

My goal for today is to replace as many negative thoughts as I can with positive thoughts. I know from experience smiling makes me feel happier than frowning, so when I encounter a negative thought, I will push it out the window and think of something good. The world is such a wonderful place, I am sure it won't be that hard.

(Re)memories

July 14, 2010

IT'S THE NIGHT BEFORE a doctor's appointment, so I am anxious and unable to focus on work. In an effort to relax, I picked up a book: *Annie Freeman's Fabulous Traveling Funeral* by Kris Radish. Normally, I don't read fiction, but something about the first paragraph and the fact the author shares her last name with a vegetable caught my attention. Besides, my period came, and I either read and write or scream out my bedroom window and freak out the neighbors.

So far, the writing is excellent. Her prose is clever and detailed without being arrogant or boring. Basically, it is the story of five women who are asked to take their friend's ashes to sites that meant very much to her. Although I am not far into the story (page 28), she has already made me think.

The main character, Katherine, recalls her recently deceased mother, not in moments they shared, but by the scents she associated with her: Dial soap, Avon perfume, garlic, and tide. She reflects, "What you remember ... is not what they think you will remember. It is often not." In other words, we cannot control what other people remember about us and vice versa.

(RE)MEMORIES

Last night, while trying to braid my hair, I remembered for the first time in decades my grandmother used to spend hours braiding my hair. I would sit on the floor in front of her, and she would brush and smooth my hair, then slowly plait it, as she called it. While she was working, she would tell me stories about her girlhood, and I was eager to listen, even though I had heard those stories so many times I had memorized them. It is a tender memory and one I may not have recovered had I not been trying to braid my own hair.

I wonder, then, where was that memory all this time? Why is it still there? Why could I recall it when I struggle to remember where I put my marriage certificate, even though I just held it in my hand a month ago?

This recollection also makes me think more about my interactions with others, especially the young people in my life. What will they remember about me when they are grown up with families of their own? Of course, I cannot control it and wouldn't want to.

I am often surprised (and surprise others) by what people remember about me that I have forgotten. A couple of summers ago, not long after I had moved back to the Valley, a man started talking to me at the mall as I sat on a bench waiting for Jim. He knew my name and recalled many things we had done together. We were "best friends" in college, he said. Sadly, I couldn't remember him at all. I tried so hard to match his face or his voice or his recollections with my memories and kept coming up empty. It wasn't until later that night I remembered talking to him at the college bookstore, where he worked and where I spent a lot of time and all of my extra grant money. But best friends? I don't remember it that way at all.

Memories are like writing in a way. (Published writing like blogs and stuff, that is.) Once you have put it out there, you have no control over how people interpret it. I can't control the impression that you have of me. You could think I am selfish, insightful, playing the victim, boring, insincere, crude, brilliant, talented, or none of the above. Of course, I accept those consequences when I publish. I hope that the ethos I construct represents me well, but I can't be sure of that, and I don't I want to be.

Certainly, our experiences and beliefs impact the way we remember things. Our value systems filter the info we take in. Studies of eyewitness testimony reveal that there are as many ways to remember a crime as there are witnesses, which is why eyewitness testimony is increasingly becoming less valuable in courts of law.

A study discussed on NPR a couple of weeks ago explored this trend. People were asked to write about the Challenger Explosion just two days after it happened. They were given the task to describe where they were when they found out about it. Decades later they were asked to recall those moments. All of them misremembered. But, remarkably, when confronted with their own written memories, they refused to accept their current memory was false.

Given all of this, though, does that mean all of my memories are fictional? That somehow I have invented my own past? Surely, some of what I remember really did happen. But what if it didn't? Does it matter?

In some ways it does matter. If we feel we have been wronged, and we haven't, then it can have consequences for the person we blame. In addition, if we remember a time or a person in a way that is too rose-colored, then we can have real problems when trying to understand who we are today.

However, how am I to know if what I remember is what actually happened? Do photographs always tell the whole story? What if my version of an event is different than someone else's?

In any case, memory is tricky. It's never clear cut, and it is often unreliable.

I am not going to spend the night questioning my childhood memories, though. In fact, I sometimes take solace in memories of that long ago time when I felt love unconditionally. When my Pap would carry me off to bed after an all-night John Wayne movie marathon, my long, bony legs dangling over the side of one of his strong arms. I can see that image clearly in my head, but I know it is not a memory. It is a movie in my mind, brought to life by family stories and my own broken remembrances. For me, it is not the exactness of memories that matter but their impressions. After all, that's all we've really got.

More Tests

July 15, 2010

JUST ROLLED IN from the RE's office and thought I would pause for an update. Basically, he told me what I already knew (everything's fine), and we started making plans for our next course of action. Sadly, it involves more tests!

He said my right tube is perfect and so are all of my other anatomical parts. The radiologist found an air bubble on the film from my HSG, but he said it was probably nothing at all to worry about. Just in case, though, he wants me to have a sonohysterogram, which involves filling my uterine cavity with saline solution and sending out sound waves to get the best picture possible of my uterus.

I guess he is just making sure, but I have to say, I am really tired of procedures. It seems every time I see him, there is something else he needs me to do. I am going to go along with it. After all, there is no reason to invest time and effort into this whole gig if there is an abnormality that could be preventing conception or could cause a miscarriage.

Meanwhile, he wants me to repeat some blood tests related to PCOS. He wants to make sure my hormone levels (male and female) and insulin levels are as good as possible. I think it is a good idea, and I welcome the knowledge to be gained from these tests.

Hubby also has to go in for a procedure. He needs to do a repeat sperm analysis. The last time most everything looked good: count (double normal levels), movement (twice as fast as average), etc. The only concern my doctor had was with the shape, or morphology, of his sperm. They are supposed to be at 14. His were at 12. He said there is nothing to worry about, really, but he thinks another test would be helpful. And, if we want, he could take Jim's sample that day and freeze it for future IUI use.

As for the future... he thinks I am an excellent candidate for IVF. I am the right age, and I am overall very healthy (my blood pressure was 116/73, for example), but he says there are steps we can take before then and we "very likely will not need future intervention."

I became very excited when I heard him say that. He says if I continue with my good health he thinks we can get pregnant on our own. The surgeries I had in May should improve our chances of conceiving naturally tremendously!

However, he said if I want we could do two things after we get the results back:

1. Do 1-2 more cycle of Clomid. Any more than that could put me at risk for developing ovarian cancer later down the road.
2. Injectable drugs, such as gonadotropins, in combination with IUI.

I told him I would think about and talk with my husband.

This is all overwhelmingly good news, and I am starting to wonder if, now that the surgeries corrected some problems, if we relax and take it easy for a few cycles if we might not be able to do it on our own. I ovulate on my own, which if you understand PCOS, you know how good that is, so maybe, just maybe we can do it.

I know I will be incapable of taking any fertility meds until December. I am teaching five classes this fall (145 students), and there is no way I can make it through a schedule like that while on crazy-making treatments, but maybe in January, we can try injectable meds.

I have briefed Jim about this, but we still need to talk about it in more detail this weekend. I am eager to hear what he thinks.

I asked my doctor if he thinks waiting until next summer to do IVF will seriously hinder our chances of conceiving. He said, "Not really. Only by a small percentage." I was relieved to hear that. My other doctor made me feel frightened when she said we needed to do this now; that we were running out of time. My doctor says 40 is really the cutoff in terms of success rates. That leaves us with three years or so to try.

Of course, the thought of keeping up this pace for that long is terrifying, but I refuse to think of it that way. One day at a time.

Meanwhile, he wants me to go on a course of antibiotics to clear up any possible infections I might have. I might take antibiotics once every five years, so I agreed with his plan.

Overall, I feel good about this news. He was very informative, and I feel I have a better handle on the situation. I wish that I could do IVF right now, but I am willing to wait until next year to re-think it. I would much rather conceive by other means than IVF. It is costly and has hazards (including failure) of its own.

Now, I wait. My period still isn't here, but I have been spotting since late last night. As soon as I see red flow, I have to call and make my appointment for the next procedure. Meanwhile, I am going to try to enjoy life. I am not really in a holding pattern, but rather in the research and development stage, which is not such a bad place to be in. I no longer feel helpless about TTC, but I know I have no control over what happens. I just hope my future includes a sweet little baby with red hair and blue eyes like my husband. Ultimately, I just long for a small voice to call me "Mama," a blessed word that I have been denied for far too long.

Fear Factor: Infertile Myrtle Style

July 18, 2010

SADLY, SO MANY of my life decisions have been motivated by fear. Fear of the unknown. Fear of failure. Fear of embarrassment. Fear of winning, even. In an effort to limit the amount of power fear has over my actions and inactions, this summer I have committed to doing things that scare me. Today, I am revisiting my list and adding to it.

I became a chicken when I was a little girl. I heard the same loud voices telling me I should be afraid of XYZ because it could: (1) kill me, (2) kill someone else, (3) hurt me, (4) hurt someone else, (5) make me look bad, (6) make someone else look bad, etc. While I will admit I had a choice as to whether or not to listen to those voices, it is pretty well known that if you keep hearing the same messages over and over again you start to believe them.

An example:

Around age 16, when everyone else was getting their driver's licenses, I was not. My parents repeatedly said I would never be able to drive because I am girl, I can't drive, and I can't learn to drive. The main message: you'll kill someone. So, I did not get my driver's license until the age of 34. You read that right. I had my Ph.D. and had been teaching college for more than a decade by the time I learned to drive and get my driver's license. It took incredible psychological will to do that. I read every book I could on how to overcome driving phobia, but what I needed most was to prove that when I got behind the wheel of the car no one was going to die, including me.

In the end, Jim helped me the most because he taught me how to drive. Learning to drive is another example of me over-thinking things. I made it more complicated than it is. Now, I love driving, and have done many long road trips alone and with my incredibly wonderful (but terribly car sick) cats.

However, and I am the first to admit there is almost always a "however," there have been times when I was told I could not do something, and I just didn't believe the hype. Going to college, for example. My parents, friends, etc. told me I would never get into college and I would surely never graduate. I didn't believe them, and I ended up graduating from college three times.

Therefore, I wonder, what makes someone believe or disbelieve a positive or negative message? Are some people prone to being afraid?

Certainly, I have seen my own fears realized: my house burned down, I have had two children die, etc. But other fears, fear of drowning, fear of ghosts, have not materialized. Part of the problem is I have let fears rule my life, which has held me back from so much.

This summer I have conquered the following fears:

1. I had reproductive surgery. I was told to have it in 2005, but I was too afraid to go under the knife. I faced my fears and did it for the greater good. I made it out just fine, and I am glad I did it.
2. I went swimming far out into the ocean. I am a good swimmer, but swimming in the ocean is far different. But with Jim's support, I took a dive and there I went. Yeah, I got beat up a bit, but I did it, and I can't wait to do it again.
3. I climbed out onto Table Rock. It is far, far above the ground, but out I went. I even looked over the side. It is the best way to truly see wv hills.
4. I went through the boxes from the fire. I relied on help to get me through it, but I dug right in there and faced each crumbling piece, and I even opened Nicholas' stash. It was painful, but well worth it!
5. I had a long talk with my husband about problems I have with his family. I was so scared that I was shaking, but it came out better than I thought.

6. I started a blog! I was afraid of putting my thoughts and feelings out in the public eye, but it has been the best move I could have made.
7. I went canoeing. That might not sound scary to you, but it sure was to me. A canoe tipping in murky flood water does not sound like a good time. I did it, though.

Now, for the rest of the summer, I have two more fears to conquer:

1. Jump off the side of the pool. This one probably sounds silly to you, and it even sounds silly to me until I am standing there looking into the drink. I have done this twice in my life. At around age 12 or so, I jumped off the dive into 9 ft. of water. I could not swim. My friend Kristy saved me! Then, two summers ago, after 45 minutes or more of hem-hawing and stammering, my friend Shannon got me to jump off the side of the pool. In both case, I was fine, but I am still terribly afraid of it.

The funniest part about this fear is watching little kids do it over and over again, while I am standing there shivering in my suit, too scared to even dip a toe in. I swim laps almost every day, and I can float like a cork. What am I really afraid of?

2. I want to find my sister. I have two half-sisters. We lost touch when we were children. My oldest sister lives here in Wheeling, or so I have been told. I am going to find her, call her, and see what happens. I have written her at least a dozen letters over the years, but I never had the courage to send them. What if she rejects me? What if she and I don't have anything in common? What if she hates our mother? What if...? Enough of that, I am going to track her down and see what happens.

I have six weeks to face both fears. I think I can do this.

Big Fat Goalie

July 19, 2010

I JUST CAN'T SEEM to quiet my mind lately. It seems that everywhere I turn I am reminded of the difficulties of living a sane, peaceful life, especially in America. Marriages are disrupted by affairs. Families are torn apart by lies. Personal strength is shredded by encounters with dysfunctional others. Nonetheless, we all find a way to move from point A to point B. How many of us, though, stop to ponder the meaning of our lives?

I had a chat this afternoon with an old friend. She said she feels like she has made it to where she wants to go in life, but she feels her life is stale, like she is still missing something. I suggested instead of an abrupt change, perhaps a gradual one might be more helpful in getting her moving again. I know how easy it is to be sucked up by the monotony of everyday life. There is comfort in it, but there is also a kind of soul death.

My ex-husband told me more than once he thought I would never be happy. There are times when I think he might be right, but most of the time I think we just share different worldviews. I know I will never be content with mediocre. I know I will never live my life without a goal. A life without goals gets you stuck down a blind alley at the mercy of others. No thanks, mister.

But I do get what he was saying. Perhaps I have been so focused on goal setting and achieving that I have ignored the blessings in my life. My gratitude list is getting longer, so it seems I am appreciating my life.

However, does having a goal, mean that I am ungrateful for what I already have? Is the desire to have a child asking too much?

I end with a few lines from Ellery, a Cincinnati band that really gets you in the gut:

TWO-WEEK WAIT

Remember how,
We chased it like shadows
Life was the ocean,
We wanted to swim

Hip Check

July 20, 2010

IT'S FUNNY HOW you can live in a body for 36+ years and still discover something new about it and yourself.

For years I struggled with overcoming bad body image. Sudden weight gain at puberty from the onset of Polycystic Ovarian Syndrome (PCOS) and my menstrual cycle backhanded my tomboy confidence and propelled me into the world of the hypersensitive teenage girl. It took me decades to silence my internal body-bashing monologue, and I did most of that work through writing.

Occasionally, I have days where I don't like what I see in the mirror, but on those days, I pat myself on the stomach or the thigh or whatever part doth offend and thank my body for another day of making it possible for me to enjoy the crunch of fall leaves under my feet, the feel of my cat's soft fur on my face, and the sweet taste of tomatoes fresh from my garden. It is not a perfect relationship, but my body and I get along pretty well these days.

One of the major steps I took on this road to body love involved getting to know myself better by figuring out what I appreciate about me. I love the way my toes are perfect little rounds at the end of my feet. I love my big brown, shiny eyes. I love my breasts, large and full. And I could go on and on. Given this body knowledge, it was quite a surprise to discover my hips for the first time last night.

You are probably thinking, "I have met you, girlie, and your hips are not exactly well hidden." In fact, my hips are probably my biggest body part after my butt. My thighs are certainly in the top three. I am a classic pear shape, a fact that I once hated, but have come to love. I am who I am because I am.

Anyway, I was getting ready for bed last night, and I had just pulled on my nightgown. As I smoothed it down over my hips, my hands lingered. My hips felt enormous under my touch, as though they had grown a foot on each side. However, instead of moaning at what might be weight gain, I giggled. In fact, I giggled so loud, I woke up my husband. He murmured a "you okay?" in his sleep-filled voice, and I giggled again, explaining to a man who would not hear me that I love my hips.

I got into bed and marveled at the way they spread out under me, taking up a pretty big chunk of my side of the bed. It was as though I was a baby who had just discovered her own feet. I couldn't stop looking, feeling, and enjoying my own hips.

I don't know why I had this sudden "seeing" moment. Maybe it was because I had heard a woman on the radio talking about fat people who are too psychologically blind to notice. Or maybe it was because I had just re-read my old essay, *Loving the Fat Girl*, the night before. In any case, I was enamored.

On the one hand, my lower body size can be problematic. I have trouble squishing into small spaces, like amusement park rides and airplane seats. On the other hand, I feel so comfortable with myself that those moments seem like a trivial trade off.

I realized long ago being healthy is not about a number on the scale. I have lost 100 pounds. Do I feel better at my current weight than I did then? Oh yeah. But I believe it has more to do with who I am now and not how much I weigh. Back then, I suffered from severe body hatred and anxiety. I felt like the world couldn't stop staring at the fat girl, and in fact, I was verbally abused for my weight on more than one occasion. But what I came to realize through my writing is I will never be a size 6, and I am just fine with that.

It might seem blasphemous to some of you. I mean, who wouldn't want to be thin, right? But to me, being healthy and happy and confident is not correlated to my weight in pounds. I have been miserable thin and fat and really fat. I have been happy at those weights, too.

Trust me, I am not deluding myself (or diluting myself, either). I know that obesity can be hard on the body, but I think punishing your body with one extreme weight loss regime after another and bouts of working out like a maniac for two months and then being a couch potato for six are not exactly healthy. I do right by my body most of the time by eating organic, whole foods, limiting sugars, consuming lots of fiber and good fats, avoiding most animal products, being active every day, taking it easy when necessary, nourishing my skin, caring for my spiritual self and so on.

But what I won't do is beat myself up about my cellulite-dimpled thighs or underarm jiggle. This doesn't mean I don't want to look and feel my best. What it means is that my mental wellbeing is far more important than what other people think of the size of my behind or the wiggle in my walk.

Beyond that, even though my weight has been roughly the same now for about two years, I have never felt healthier. I am rarely ever tired, I have regular periods, my blood pressure is great (117/73), my cholesterol is awesome (125 total), and all of my other markers look as good as anyone else my age (and some are even better).

Am I going to run a marathon? No. But I really don't want to. I would rather swim laps for an hour or spend the afternoon in my garden or in our canoe or hiking in the mountains than worry about whether the guy who works at the gas station thinks my waist is too small for my hips.

And that brings me back to my re-discovery. I think that I giggled so when I appreciated the fullness of my hips because I liked the feeling of their mass pressing back at me as I smoothed down my nightgown. I like knowing that I take up space in this world. That to be in my life, you have to give me room to spread out.

In the end, I lost that 100 pounds not because I was trying to get thin, but because I was trying to be healthier. The weight loss was a nice side effect of changing my diet. I kicked out foods that were making me sick and began to live in my body instead of hiding it from the world. So, fat, thin, or somewhere in between I vow to love the body I have and never again reach for a body I don't or never will. Goals are good, but not when they come at the expense of being present in the present. I am thankful every day for a body that carries me through the world. And you should be, too.

The Rhythm of Love

July 23, 2010

WE ALL BELIEVE that we know how to love. From the time we first wrap our arms around our mother's shoulders to the day we bring a blanket to our shivering spouse, we think we have a pretty good handle on what it means to love another person. It turns out, it isn't that simple.

The other day my therapist said we all believe our version of love, of what it means to love another person, is the same as everyone else's. She said there is no universal concept of love. I struggle with that idea. Surely, there must be some features that all humans recognize as love.

But then I realized like other emotions, love is relative.

For example, some people think spanking their children when they misbehave is an act of love. By helping them understand right from wrong, these parents think they are helping their children be better people, which will pay off when they are adults. It is, to them, a way of expressing love. Other people feel spanking is wrong and demonstrates anything but love to the child. Instead of teaching them how to be better humans, spanking teaches children violence is okay and people who love you sometimes physically hurt you.

It is complicated.

Understanding that love and how a person acts or speaks when he or she loves someone is relative to that person. When you realize and ACCEPT that it sure makes your life easier. In a sense, you must have faith the person you love loves you, too. Second guessing actions and words only leads to frustration and sadness. We should never allow ourselves to be mistreated, but we should give the people we love the freedom to love us in their way. Once again, I am reminded my way of being is not universal and I can learn much from allowing others to be who they are and not who I believe or hope they will be.

Is It Worth All This?

July 26, 2010

AS PART OF MY TREATMENT for infertility, my doctor prescribed a very strong course of antibiotics in order to kill off any possible infections I might have. He said not to drink alcohol while taking them, but he never told me they would make me feel like I was auditioning for a role in a zombie flick.

The nausea and vomiting is bad enough, but the extreme exhaustion and joint pain is so much worse. I couldn't figure out why I was so tired for days and days, no matter how much sleep I got the night before. And then two days ago, the joint pain started. My legs hurts so badly last night I bound them up in a comforter and heating pad. They still hurt, and I still feel tired, but I am slowly coming out of it.

I confirmed my assumption that it was the antibiotic that caused all the pain when I found a website that focused on patient testimonials associated with the drug. Some people had it even worse than I do. At least the duration was relatively short.

Is It Worth All This?

Last night, while writhing in agony (I am not exaggerating), I thought to myself, "Is having a child really worth this?" I know that most people would say that parenthood is harder than the TTC process, but I don't think it is fair to compare the two. (More on that in upcoming entries.) In any case, as I rolled around in pain, tired beyond measure, yet unable to fall asleep, I thought about all I have gone through in the many years I have been on this journey, the worst of which being the deaths of my children.

Then, I got up to get a cup of tea and poked my head into one of our spare bedrooms. I studied the light pink walls with the kitty and puppy border and butterfly curtains, remnants of the family who lived here before us, and started thinking about how different the room would look if we had a child. I intend to re-do it this fall for no other reason than I hate the color pink, but if we had a child, it would be filled with stuffed lions, a crib, a rocking chair, and... Well, the picture became clear. Instead of gulping back tears of sadness for what isn't, I smiled as I thought of what might become.

For better or for worse, I am allowing myself to dream again, to believe one day the room will be filled with a child and his or her own things. I feel I have so much to offer a child: love, optimism, thoughtfulness, a good education, and a big room where he or she could dream and play and snuggle with a Mom who allowed herself sweet moments of hope in painful, seemingly endless quest.

This week, a child will inhabit the room. My teenaged niece is coming to stay with me for the week. I am excited about her visit and the chance to spend time with her doing fun things she likes to do. As I was freshening up the room for her arrival, bittersweet feelings washed over me. The joy of anticipating her upcoming arrival, and the sadness at knowing she will go home to her Mom at the end of the week. My children would be nine and almost 19 years old. How different life would be if they had lived. But rather than see those rooms (and my life) as empty, I prefer to see them as full. Full of my hopes and dreams for a child that will come to stay.

Another Day, Another Test

July 28, 2010

HEADING OFF TO BED early tonight. I have another fertility test tomorrow. This time, my doctor is doing a sonohystogram, which means shooting saline into my uterus and taking some pics. Oh joy!

In reality, I cannot complain too much about this. At least I have insurance that will pay for it. But I dread the drive in rush hour traffic and the pain of the procedure itself.

Thankfully, I will have a companion to keep me company, which is rare for me. My niece will ride along with me, and I will enjoy her girlish chatter, taking my mind off of what I lack. It is difficult to convince myself that my life is anything but wonderful when I have so much!

In any case, I am off to bed to get some rest before the early drive. I will post an update as soon as I can. I wonder ... will it ever stop?

Approaching the Summit

July 30, 2010

AFTER A LONG WAIT, the doctor performed the sonohystogram and pronounced that everything looks great. In other words, my results indicate I am not any different than any other 36-year-old trying to conceive. This was my last test for a while.

Jim and I talk about it, and I am taking a break from fertility drugs until the holidays, when I won't be working and I can deal with mood swings ... at least without taking them out on my students... and then move on to IVF in May of next year.

I am optimistic about all of this. The test results keep indicating that things are fine, and I am under excellent care. It is the waiting that is the hardest part, as Tom Petty says.

But lately I have been reflecting on the power of waiting. All the good things I have in my life right now I had to wait for: getting a job in the Valley, buying a house, getting PhD, marrying Jim, etc. That doesn't mean I wasn't working towards them along the way, but there was an element of waiting involved. It took me 12 years to find a way to move back to the Valley, 15 years to buy a house, 16 years to marry Jim, 10 years to get the PhD. And while I have been trying since Nicholas died in 2001 to have a baby, nine years is a relatively short period of time compared to my other dreams. And having a healthy child certainly trumps all else.

So, I just need to relax and let nature take its course for a while. I have done all that I can do for now. If no baby by next May, then I will throw some elbow grease into it and see what science has to offer. I will keep on trying to conceive, but I am going to give myself a break and know that waiting for something so wonderful is the least that I can do.

Meanwhile, I am going to enjoy my last afternoon with my niece. It has been nice having her around. She has reminded me of how joyful it can be to have a child in your life and of the difficulties of shepherding a teen. There are pitfalls along the way, but rewards to be had in spades. I hope I am up to the challenge if I am ever given the chance to bring a child home.

August 2010

Be Who You Are

August 1, 2010 at 4:26 pm

AFTER A PARTICULARLY challenging canoe trip around Wheeling Island, I felt frustrated and somewhat depressed. I was already feeling a little blue after dropping off my niece the night before, so my not-so-super boat ride pushed me over into Annoyed Land, which is not a great place to be—ever. Right in the middle of feeling sorry for myself, I looked up to see an inspirational message on the bulletin board in front of the school near my house: "Be who you are, and do that well." I smiled, thanking the universe once again for shoving a message down my throat just when I needed it most.

I like canoeing. Being out on the water in a human-powered craft is relaxing and exciting, especially when the waterway is swollen with rainwater or filled with speedboats and river barges. I am not an expert canoer. In fact, I still get confused about on which side of the boat I need to paddle to get it to go where I want it to go. But I accept that about me, and I tend to giggle a lot when I start rowing the boat in a circle. It is not that I don't help out, but I am not as strong as most other passengers and I do have an impaired sense of direction.

Not everyone appreciates my paddling deficiency, and it causes tension. Generally speaking, I am chided and eventually yelled at.

Not only does it make me feel like an incompetent buffoon, but I also feel sad and angry. Sad because I feel like I am being bullied and angry because I am not the world's best canoer, I don't want to be the world's best canoer, and everyone who knows me knows that.

All of that said, however, I started thinking about who I am and what I like and don't like. I have had trouble all of my life with figuring out who I am and what I value. I enjoy trying new activities, food, etc. because I never know when I am going to find something new that I like. And I don't mind at all doing things with other people just because it is what they like to do. I don't have to love something to spend time with someone I love doing what they like to do. To clarify, an example.

If left to my own devices, I would not go fishing. I have never enjoyed fishing, but I have gone many, many times in my life. I have been night fishing and ice fishing and fly fishing. I like to go because it gives me a chance to spend time with people I care about who do like fishing. I like being in nature, too, so it is not a bad way to spend the day. I dislike the heat, biting bugs, and trudging through mud, but there are worst ways to share my time with people I love.

I am not a fisherwoman.

That said, I have been struggling for quite some time to figure out who I am. It sounds simple. I am a writer, a professor, a wife, a daughter, a cat lover, a yoga enthusiast, a singer, a gardener, a homeowner, a taxpayer, a West Virginian, a licensed driver, a woman, a vegetarian, a swimmer, a coffee drinker, a non-smoker, a 36 year old, and the list goes on.... But what does all that mean? What do those labels tell me (or you) about who I am? After all, isn't who I am mediated through cultural lenses? In some countries, I would be considered a true beauty for my round butt and big arms. In other cultures (my own, for example), fatness is not on the list of attractive qualities for most people. Even in my own community, some of my qualities are interpreted differently. The girl who makes my cappuccino in the mornings loves that I do yoga because she teachers yoga. My Dad thinks that I am a hippie weirdo for enjoying the exact same activity.

And so I wonder is there an essential ME? A ME that transcends cultural constructs? A ME that is not tethered to societal expectations? If so, how can I figure out who I AM? AND be the best at that?

I am currently reading *Eat, Pray, Love*. I came to the memoir late, partly because I generally stay away from popular memoirs. The authors often do not interrogate their lives in enough depth to suit my taste, and I come away from most bestsellers disappointed. I began reading Eat, Pray, Love at the request of my niece, and I am surprised at the quality of writing. It is interesting, introspective, humorous, and well written. In case, you don't know, Gilbert takes readers along with her on her personal journey in search of enlightenment. She travels to Italy, India, and then to Indonesia. I am not finished with it yet, so don't worry, I won't spoil the ending for you.

I bring the book up in this entry because of what Gilbert has to offer readers in terms of trying to find the divine inside us all. And I suppose that is really who I AM: divine, of God, of the universe, a small part of a much, much larger whole. Knowing that and living it out daily is a serious challenge. Garret discusses this near impossibility as well, as she struggles with her own inner demons, especially with her ego, which disrupts her meditation attempts and prevents her from discovering her own connection to divinity.

In the end, I guess the best way to get to know who I am is to get to know God.

Most people I know approach God through organized religion. As I have noted here before, that has never been my path. I have tried to find God that way over and over and over again and found failure and an even deeper yearning in almost every attempt. Other people approach the divine through prayer. And still others, like

Gilbert, approach God through meditation. In other words, there are many ways of getting in touch with the Higher Power, and therefore, it seems, with your true self, free of ego and cultural trappings.

I truly expected to write about who I think I am in this blog entry. I thought I would write about the gifts I bring to the world, but it turns out that I have only seen a glimpse of those things. In reality, I only know a little of who I am and most of that identity is defined by my relationship with others and not with mySelf. It would appear, dear readers, that my quest to have a child has revealed yet another layer of inquiry and another opportunity to dig deeper into the mysteries of my mind and of the universe itself. Into the woods, actual and metaphorical, I go!

Enjoying the NOW

August 3, 2010 at 11:49 am

I SPENT MOST of the day yesterday with my friend and her soon-to-be-four little girl. We had so much fun playing, going for a walk, and swinging on the swings. It really made me see what I am missing, but thankfully, I didn't dwell on the lack, but instead, I stayed focused on the moment.

One of my biggest improvements since I started blogging this past March is that I have become more mindful. That is, I can more easily stay in the moment than ever before. Instead of thinking about how much I wish a certain moment would last or what I will do when the day is done or other unproductive chatter, my mind is calmer and more focused on the present.

Of course, there were fleeting thoughts of grief throughout the day. At one point, I was carrying her because she had grown tired of walking. She put her hand on my face and her head on my shoulder. The tenderness of the gesture and how much I long for such an everyday moment made me push back tears.

But for most of the day, I enjoyed their company and was able to be in the NOW and not in the THEN or SOMEDAY. Why ruin a lovely afternoon by focusing on lack?

Being present in the present has become a theme for my life this summer. It is challenging, and like most difficult actions, requires practice to master. In addition to yoga and intentional walking, I try to practice being present through meditation, which is harder than it sounds.

According to Sogyal Rinpoche, a Tibetan llama and author of the *Tibetan Book of Living and Dying*, there are three main ways to meditate, and he recommends combing them all.

Focus on an object that has considerable meaning to you, such as a crystal or a flower or a religious statue or painting.

Focus on a mantra with deep meaning for you. There are many mantras, including Om, which is the generic mantra used on tv shows in which yoga-doing characters are featured. LOL

Focus on the breath. By concentrating on the breath, then you can focus on the now.

I have tried two and three, usually with good effect. I will try the first one tonight. I am not sure what object I will focus on, but I will find something. I am thinking of using an object from the natural world, something that is alive, but I could just as easily focus on this lovely statue of a black cat my friend got me for Christmas. I love cats and revere them, so this just might help me get in touch with the divine.

Meditation can be powerful. It is a way to find peace and to find God. In my case, I need a way to quiet my mind. It gets so loud in here sometimes with plans, writing ideas, conversation snippets, and memories that I need something to shut it down just for a little while.

Sometimes I feel like I am throwing everything I find at the problems in my life: yoga, meditation, blogging, talking, texting, walking, boating, etc. Some things work and some things don't. In the end, I think this has been a summer of experimentation and expansion. I have learned to be more mindful, to be patient, and to love myself even more. Will all of these efforts lead to bringing a child home? I don't know. And for right now, I am okay with that.

Reunited . . . and It Feels So Good?

August 5, 2010 at 5:41 pm

REUNION SEASON is upon us. Family reunions. Class reunions. Friends reunions. And so on. Summer is the time of get togethers and traveling together and getting ourselves together. It is no wonder, then, that many of my conversations lately have turned to reuniting with others and dealing with the subsequent consequences.

The high school class a year ahead of mine is getting together next weekend for its 20th reunion. Yeah, it is been almost twenty years since my high school days. It doesn't seem like it has been that long ago, but that is what the calendar says. They have kindly invited graduates from other years to attend, and some of us are, but I have declined. Reunions of any kind fill me with ambivalence, as I am sure they do most people.

In some ways, I would like to go. I knew some of those people for thirteen years or longer, as we struggled from kindergarten through high school. Some of them were wonderful friends. Some were bitter enemies. Over the years, though, they have all kind of blended together to become people. Just people. We are thirtysomethings getting by in a society that isn't all that unlike the one that we plowed through for much of our school years. The past decade has been quite similar to the 80s for some of us: lack of jobs, depression, etc. As young people we were taught to "Say No to Drugs," call McGruff the Crime Dog if we see danger, avoid drinking stuff with Mr. Yuck on the front, not have unprotected sex for fear of AIDS, not drink and drive because some people will get MADD, not talk to strangers or we might get abducted and murdered like Adam, not eat our Halloween candy until it was X-rayed for razor blades, and to beware of the Russians because they were going to nuke us.

But now, we have families of our own to care for and car payments to make and food to buy. No longer children, those of us who graduated on the cusp of the 1990s face struggles that we could not have imagined then. From what I understand, many of us have been divorced and re-married a few times. We have kids and stepkids and even grandchildren. We go to therapy, and some of us take our kids, too. Some of us lost our houses in the mortgage bust. Others of us lost our retirement savings, then, too.

At the same time, we have quite a bit to celebrate. Today's thirtysomethings are working hard for charities, making sure our kids get good educations, and serving our communities. We aren't slouches, as some people would like to believe. Us Gen-Xers do contribute to our world. Despite being handed an economy in the dumper and a political system in meltdown, we have managed to keep it together enough to get by, and in the end, that is about all a group of people can really do.

So far, my thirties have been the best decade of my life. I am established in my career, make enough money to afford a nice home (and pay back my student loans; PhDs ain't cheap), feel confident about who I am, share my life with amazing, caring people, and have the opportunity to devote a big portion of my life to things I love: writing, my animals, my family and friends, and of course, my husband.

My school years, however, were far different, as I am sure they were for most people. I had trouble getting along well with others. I had problems with self-esteem and with coping with poverty. I lived in an abusive home, and my role models were poor, for the most part. These factors, along with a hormone-trigged weight problem, came together to create an unhappy child and a severely depressed adolescent. It is no wonder I had trouble making and keeping friends.

For years, I looked back on my school years with regret, anger, and sadness. I hated some of my classmates. Rather than see us all as mixed up young people, I saw them as bullies. They hated me. They mocked me. They teased me. While they did do those things, I failed to see what role I played in these troubling interactions. It took me more than a decade to come to terms with those demons and to own my part in those desperately sad years.

I do not excuse their cruelty, but I also do not excuse my own bad behavior. I feel sympathy for my young, battered self, and I can certainly see why I acted out the way I did, but it is no wonder I had trouble making friends and keeping them. I was self-centered, annoying, and just as mean.

What I have realized is those high school labels—nerds, jocks, preps, dirtbags, sluts, druggies, band geeks—fall away as the years march on. It becomes harder and harder as we roar through our twenties and drift into our thirties to maintain such strict definitions for others and especially for ourselves. And all of those things that seemed to matter most back then (hair styles, clothes, parents' occupations) don't matter at all now. (Pay attention nieces, nephews, and especially my students.) What matters now are what should have mattered all along: compassion, honesty, humor, personal ethics, commitment, loyalty, love. But we were just kids. What did we know?

For years, I dreaded visiting my parents. I moved away for graduate school in 1996 and could never imagine moving back to the Valley. I had such painful memories of this place. But after awhile, the call of home was too hard to ignore, and I moved back two years ago. To my surprise, some of the people I barely new in high school (or thought hated me or I hated them) have become my good friends. I realized that quite a bit of that high school drama was just that, drama, and most of it created in my head. In fact, some of what I remembered in high school no one else seemed to even notice. We build things up so big in our own minds, and it causes unnecessary pain. And even for me it is hard to believe after a summer of visits from friends from all over the country that I was once a sad, frightened young girl who felt left out and hated by her peers.

But given that this is an entry in MY blog, you know I have to add some funny memories to keep it real. What I am about to relate caused me terrible embarrassment at the time, but I can't help but laugh about them now. I hope you do too!

In kindergarten I told everyone I had a real, live kangaroo at home. I didn't really believe that I did (I did become a writer, you know), but everyone thought that I was convinced of it and my moniker as fabulist was henceforth assigned.

In first grade I was busted for being creative. I got bored and stapled crayons to my notebook and got whatever the primary grade equivalent to detention is.

In fifth grade, my period started, and I gained more than 40 lbs. Half of it was boobs and the other half pimples.

In sixth grade, I jumped off the dive into nine feet of water. I couldn't swim. A skinny girl in my class jumped in to save me, and she doesn't even remember it. It must have been hilarious to see this twiggy girl carrying this chubby girl on her back to the safety of the poolside. (I love her for that and have thanked her more than once in recent years.)

Throughout my entire school year, I got in trouble for talking, but in seventh grade, I got busted for chewing gum and was forced to stand out in the hallway during class change with gum stuck on my nose. (I know I am not the only one. Don't judge.)

In eighth grade two chicks caught my hair on fire at a thuse. That Aquanet sure goes up fast! I didn't even know I was on fire until they started hugging me to put out the flames.

At an Awards Day ceremony in ninth grade, I caught my pump heel on the bleacher steps and went flying through the air, landing in the middle of the basketball court with my stirrup pants ripped. Everyone in the entire school saw my pink underwear. (Thankfully, my friend sewed them back together for me in the locker room. I love her to this day for that!)

In tenth grade, I knocked my friends tooth out with a battery. What? We were bored and trying to see how many AAs we could toss into her sweatshirt. I missed! (She forgave me for it, thankfully.)

I was in many plays in high school. In eleventh grade, I was in a play with a bunch of girls. We had to wear black body suits. Seriously. One of those girls was absolutely kind to me. Since then, we have become good friends. She often says it is like we were separated at birth. I am flattered by that every time!

I dropped out of high school in March of my senior year. I was pregnant. I repeated my senior year and graduated in 1993. That year, I met a girl who became and remains my BFF and a boy I instantly fell in love with and would have sold my soul to marry if I wasn't still in shock when I met him.

In the end, what I have learned in the many years since I turned my tassel to the other side of my cap is that nothing is forever, we all play a role in our misery, people are people are people, and we must love each other in this life. I know it is hard sometimes not to judge others. I have that problem sometimes, too, but I have learned that we are all the same: thirtysomethings trying to get by in a hard knock world. But there is so much beauty to be had if only we look for it. Those high school cliques have long ago dissolved, and all that remains is humanity. We are a bunch of West Virginia hillbillies living life just like anyone else.

Even still, when a cute boy I had a huge crush on in high school sends me a "Hello" message on Facebook or a girl I have been missing since the eleventh grade bumps into me at Kroger, I get excited, and memories–good and bad–come flooding back. Suddenly, we are 15 years old again, but this time I am what I wish I had been all those years ago: compassionate, open, loving. We are all fellow travelers on this road of life. We should be good to each other.

So, those of you going to the reunion next weekend, enjoy yourselves! And don't let memories of high school dramas get in the way of getting to know that girl who sat next to you in biology or those boys who used to have pickles races down the wall in the Commons. Oh, and don't forget to say, "It's okay" before you head into the bathroom. You never know who might be smokin' in there. Love you guys!

Finding a Focus

August 8, 2010 at 8:47 pm

HEALERS OF ALL STRIPES, including MDs right here in the states, have long advocated the use of meditation as a tool on the road to wellness. Not only does meditation help alleviate stress, it helps those who practice it to focus on and trust their own thoughts. I know that some folks think that meditation is some kind of new-agey, hippie thing (and it is!), but in reality, it is one of many options for finding balance and strength in life. However, meditation sounds a whole lot easier than it is.

If you read my blog regularly and/or if you talk to me in real life, then you know that I talk–a lot! Well, imagine, then, how loud it is in my head. I am constantly thinking. Not just planning what I will do next, but reflecting on what just happened and what happened decades ago. I am a thinking machine. And people, that ain't no good.

I think so much that I can't get a word in edgewise, and it is my head! And wow, I have a really hard time getting quiet (in person and in thought). Yoga has helped me get quiet quicker and so has meditation, but I still struggle with meditating. I needed a focus, and I finally found one: Ganesh.

I have mentioned my elephant-headed deity here before, and in the past week or so I have done more research on him to try to determine if he is the right focus for me. Now, don't freak out on me here. I am not saying that I worship Ganesh or that I pray to him. Rather, I use what he represents as a point of focus for my meditations.

Ganesh is known for destroying obstacles. People look to him for help with trying to overcome something. Obviously, I have things to overcome, including my restless mind.

My first attempts at more concentrated meditation sounded a little something like this:

> *Om. Om. It feels hot in here. Om. Om. Maybe I should turn a fan on. Om. Om. Am I sitting up straight enough? Om. Om. Is there a cat in the room? I wonder if it is Toby or Ginger? Om. Om. I wish it was darker in here. I can see light coming through my eyelids. Om. Om. Man, I wish I would have had more coffee. Maybe even a sandwich. I wonder if I still have a half a sandwich in the fridge? Om. Om. I really need to concentrate here. Om. Om. Maybe if I put a pillow under my butt that will help. Om. Om. Oh great, now I have to pee.*

But I don't give up. I keep going, concentrating on my breath, mantra and breaking down obstacles. Before too many more Oms, I am relaxed completely.

Meditation is a wonderful tool. I suggest that you give it a shot if you haven't already.

Preparing for Tomorrow

August 10, 2010 at 4:22 pm

I DON'T REALLY HAVE time to be blogging. I am on a deadline for a book I am writing, and it has nothing to do with this blog. However, I have something I need to get off my chest.

Tomorrow is my daughter Samantha's 19th birthday. It is hard to imagine that I could be a mother of a 19 year old. I try to imagine sometimes what my life would be like if she would have lived, and there is really no way of doing that. I have no idea who she would be or what she would have become. I have reflected on that in previous entries, but I really can't fathom how different my world would be if my little girl would have survived.

I promised her that if I ever moved back to the Valley that I would visit her on her birthday. Tomorrow will make my fourth year in a row of keeping that promise. Even before I moved back, I tried to make every effort to come into town on her special day. It is a bittersweet moment for me, always. Last year, I took a big bouquet of pink roses and baby's breath and laid them on her grave. (And, of course, so my grandma wouldn't get jealous, I placed a dozen red ones on her grave, which is right next door.) I sat there in the quiet of the cemetery reflecting on the previous year, loss, love, and happiness. Yes, happiness.

At that moment, sitting there amidst the graves of my most beloveds (daughter, grandmother, grandfather) I realized that they are gone from this world. There is nothing I can do to bring them back. There is nothing I can say to change anything that has come before. Instead, I spent the last part of my visit with them recalling good times. My grandmother telling me dirty jokes (Wanna hear a dirty joke? Two pigs fell in the mud. Wanna here a dirtier joke? Two pigs fell in the mud and three came out.); my grandfather making me special pancakes with sugary crusts and homemade syrup (Here, let me cut that up for you.); and my little girl's giggle, so sweet and honest from her chubby mouth.

Tomorrow's entry, like any time I write about my children, will be a reflection on love and loss. I have written about her death before but this time, I will tell Samantha's story as best I can. Her story is my story. My story is her story. And both are never ending.

To My Daughter, On Her Birthday

August 11, 2010 at 1:55 am

NINETEEN YEARS AGO at this very moment, I was looking out the window of the camper trailer where I lived with my first husband wondering when my baby would be born and hoping it would be soon. I remember that it was 12:30 in the morning because he said, "It is 12:30 in the morning, and you should come to bed." I wasn't tired. I was excited. I was anxious. I was scared. But I wasn't tired. Eighteen hours later, my daughter, Samantha Christine, would be born.

I got pregnant just days before my seventeenth birthday. I found out, ironically, while at a doctor's appointment to get birth control pills. When the nurse asked me if I wanted to keep the positive test as a memento, I looked at her with what must have been shell-shocked eyes and said, "No. God. No."

My then-boyfriend tried to convince me to have an abortion. His brilliant plan was to punch me in the stomach when I wasn't expecting it, and I would have a miscarriage and all would be well. I thought he was just scared of becoming a Dad. I obviously gave him too much credit.

When I refused his beat-me-until-I-miscarry plan, he recommended an abortion. We go to the nearest city, I get the abortion, we come back, we tell no one. For a week or so that seemed like a good idea. I even called the clinic and set up an appointment, but when the day came, I backed out. We were in the car somewhere between home and the interstate, my purse full of Advil and maxipads, when I began crying. I could not go through with it. I could not take this life. He pulled over and eventually said we would somehow get through it together. We went on into the city. We had lunch. We allowed ourselves, just a little, to get used to the idea that we were going to have a baby.

We hid it from our families for a couple of months. I continued working at the ice cream store. He continued working at the fast food place. He was five years older than me. I was a high school senior. I had all but stopped going to school by that time. I skipped just about daily, pretending to ride the bus, but instead taking a detour through the neighborhood to where he lived with his sister. We would spend the days warm and cozy in his bed those early winter months, until I had to go home and he had to go to work.

We argued, but it never seemed more than what one would expect. I never felt incredibly loved by him, but I did feel like we might be on the right road.

When I started to show, we realized we had to do something. I had been spending most of my time in my bedroom reading every baby book I could get my hands on. And it became pretty obvious that there would be no way to continue hiding my growing belly.

I turned to the Department of Human Services. They had to know what to do, and they sure did. The social worker told me I had two choices: go to the Florence Crittenton Home for Unwed Mothers or marry the baby's father. Neither of those options seemed like a good choice. I asked if they would be willing to help me start up a life, just the baby and me, the way I had seen so many other single mothers in my community do. She repeated her answer. I walked out crying and stunned.

My choices, then, were to live in a home with other pregnant girls or marry a man I had known for less than six months. While everyone reading this (and even the chic writing it) can understand that I did get pregnant, and I did know what I was doing at the time, I hope you all will also understand just why those choices were really no choices at all. Rather than live in what was basically a homeless shelter for knocked up teens, I decided that my best option was to marry my unborn baby's father. I did love him, and we could certainly make it work over time. Shotgun weddings are not a new social invention.

Later that night, I made him ask my father if he could marry me. At first my Dad said no. I had to graduate from high school first. (Kudos to Dad.) Nervously, my almost-fiancé asked again, adding, "You are going to be a grandfather." To say that my Dad was angry would be inadequate. I think if he could have tossed us both through a wall he would have, but instead, he told us to get out. And so we did. We walked the four miles to his sister's house on the iciest roads I have ever slid on. But I was so excited! I was getting married. I did not have to live at home ever again! (Once again, I was wrong.)

We got married on February 19 (or was it February 17?). I was almost five months pregnant. My tummy bulges just slightly in the wedding pictures. I am in a blue dress with black pumps, all borrowed. There are four people there: both sets of our parents. The now-husband tried to pick up his ex-girlfriend on the way over to the church, but I was resolutely against it. (Silly me.)

We had no money for a honeymoon, so we went to a cafeteria (complete with roaches) for lunch, and then he went to work. Yes, that's right friends, he went to work the day we got married. While he was gone that night, I sat on the twin bed in his room and painted our wedding bands with nail polish to ensure that they would not turn our fingers green.

If you think I am being unnecessarily grim about the whole affair, I assure you I am not. There was nothing romantic about that night. I was happy to marry him, that is unmistakable when you look at the photos (all lost to the house fire), but no girl would be happy that her husband went to work (at a fast food restaurant!) on the night they got married.

I tried to stay in school for a while. I remember doing trig homework while Samantha kicked inside me. But I was bored with school before the pregnancy and marriage. It held no charm at all for me after. In early March, I walked in to my high school and dropped out, continuing a long-standing family tradition, but I had gotten farther than anyone else in the family. And I had a new title, "Emancipated Minor."

The pregnancy was wonderful. I loved being pregnant. Even though I gained nearly 80 lbs by the time I gave birth, I was never happier than when I shared my body with this little soul. I would talk to her every night, reassuring her that her life would be as good as Mommy could make it.

Meanwhile, my new husband was not so happy. He was struggling to find work that paid more than minimum wage. He had no education beyond a GED, so the outlook was poor. We decided to move to a little town in Ohio, not far from our families, but closer to his friends. We lived in a small, but nice apartment for a while. Then, we had to move because we could not afford the rent increase once our baby was born. My welfare check and food stamps would not cover the rent and put food on the table, so we rented his parents' camper trailer and put it on a lot by the highway.

The camper trailer, the one who's window I was peering out of the night before Samantha was born, was one room (not including the bathroom). It had running water and a stove. The table folded down to make a bed. What it did not have was a fan. I was eight months pregnant. It was summer. I drank a lot of water and ate a lot of ice cream from the Dairy Queen next door. I would have drank beer at the bar on the other side, but I was pregnant and all.

It was a miserable way to live. I didn't have my driver's license. I had no money. I had no hope. All I had was this incredible life growing inside me, and a wonderful cat named Lucky, who I adopted from a yard sale down the street. My husband had grown angrier. Obviously, he felt trapped. He hoped that my intelligence or my singing ability would get us out of extreme poverty, but neither one panned out until much later.

To My Daughter, On Her Birthday

My water broke at Noon on August 11. I applied make up (I was 17!), packed a bag, and headed to my mother's house. I went for a walk, fearing that they would confine me to a bed at the hospital. Finally, the contractions were too close together to put off, and I found myself being wheeled into the delivery room in agonizing pain. I refused pain medication, preferring a natural birth. Just six hours later, at 6:02 pm, Samantha Christina was born. She weighed 8 lbs and 12 oz and was 22 inches long. She was perfect and beautiful and wonderful. I was scared.

They put her in my arms. I looked into her little red face peering out from beneath her mint green hat, and I was overcome with absolute joy and panic. I had never held a newborn before. I had never fed, bathed, changed, or touched a baby, and here I was holding my own. I was her caretaker.

I breastfed her and rocked her and told her that I loved her. Inside, I was trembling with fear and exhaustion.

Not long after we were released from the hospital, her father decided to go south for a while and live with his uncle and his family. He could get a good job there, save up money, and then come back and get us when he had enough money to rent an apartment. He came back to visit me for my 18th birthday. He brought me a winter coat and a book of poems, Coleridge, which he bought in Philippe. It was old, 1927. I was touched. He was not a reader, but he knew that I loved to read and that I needed a coat.

He spent a few days with us. We had moved in with my parents for a while. Then, when it was time to leave, I begged him not to go. He said he had to because he had no money, and he could not handle her, pointing to Samantha. I cried. But he left the next day.

Just a few weeks later, we had rented an apartment across town from my parents. He moved back and got his job back at the fast food place. On November 22, 1991, he killed our daughter.

I have explained what happened to the best of my knowledge in other essays, but I will summarize it here once again. Somehow repeating it weakens its power, makes it less devastating, but unbearable pain will never be bearable no matter how much you cut it down with words, alcohol, or whatever feeble weapon you choose.

According to him and the police who investigated, he went in to the room where Samantha was crying, picked her up, and shook her to death. Later, he would tell me he "snapped," but I really do not know. I was making him dinner when he killed her. A simple act of cooking a meal for my husband, pork chops, Rice-a-Roni, and corn. Then, he put her back in her bed and came back into the kitchen, assuring me that she was now asleep, and he ate his dinner. Really. He ate his fucking dinner!

Later, we went to bed and tried to have sex, but he said he was too tired. I got up to see if she needed an extra blanket. When I touched her tiny hand, it was cold. And I knew, in my mother's heart I knew, that she was dead. Before I ever turned on the light to see her grey face and half opened eyes, I knew she was dead. I knew she would never breathe again. But in my mother's heart, I knew I had to try. I pulled her up out of her bed and tried performing mouth to mouth. I put her aside, put on my shoes, made him run with me out the apartment door and into the street, screaming all the way, "My baby! Somebody save my baby!"

I was already out of my mind as I blew my breath into her lifeless body. I was already out of my mind as I raced into the emergency room begging the nurses to help me, help her. I was already so far out of my mind when I tried to jump from the third floor parking lot into the street below after they told me she was gone.

Within 24 hours my now ex-husband would be in jail, pending trial, arrested for her murder. My little girl's murder.

But this not a story about him. This is not a story about how is family and so many other people from my hometown treated me like I was her murderer long after he went to prison under his own admission of guilt. No, this is not about them. It is about her.

To My Daughter, On Her Birthday

This is a post about my little girl, Samantha. She would be nineteen years old today. Instead, she is in the ground. She was three and a half month olds when her life was taken. She could smile and giggle. She could make beautiful baby noises. She could roll over. She could hold her own bottle.

She could not defend herself. And I could not defend her either. Unseen monsters are the worst kind.

Later today, when the sun comes up, I will go to the floral shop and buy the biggest bunch of pink roses I can find. I will get in my car and drive to the cemetery where she is buried. She shares a plot with my beloved grandfather. She sleeps eternally next to my dear grandmother and most of her family. I will remember, as I did last year, that these people are my adopted family, but they loved me far more than my biological family ever did. I will reaffirm how glad I am that my daughter shares the Earth with them. They took care of me. They will take care of her.

I have wondered if her father ever stops to visit her. He served seven and a half years for her murder, which he never once said he was sorry for. He apologized to me the day of his arrest. Crying, he kept saying over and over again in a rapid, frightened voice, "I'm so sorry." At the time, I did not know why, not knowing that he had killed her. Later, I would replay that moment over and over again, realizing that he was sorry he was going to jail, that he was sorry he had taken something from me, but he was not sorry he had taken her life. I wonder, but never for more than a moment, if he is sorry now. Does he remember her birthday? Does he go through the pain I do, almost every day of my life, because I miss my little girl so much?

After an hour or two of sitting with her, I will get up off the ground and call my husband, Jim. I will tell him I am okay. He will try to understand. I will get in my car, wishing more than anything on Earth that she was sitting next to me, now a teenage girl, so that I could look over at her and say, "Happy Birthday, Samantha! I love you." Instead, I say those words out the car window and drive away, leaving her there, as I have now for nineteen years.

The pain has definitely receded. I no longer wake up at night crying about her (at least not more than a few times a year). But I miss her still. I miss her most when I see pictures of my friends' kids at their Homecoming dances or graduations. I know, though, that nothing can bring her back. Nothing can make it so that she can live her life. And nothing will ever make it possible for me to hear her say the one word I have longed for since August 11, 1991, "Mama."

Nearly two decades later, I sit alone in my bedroom, one of three in this 1920's house I bought last year. My husband is working, and I am writing. Geographically, I am closer to that time period than I have been in years, but in every other way the distance is greater than I can even take in.

I went back to high school and finished my senior year. I went on to college and earned my degree in three years, then a Master's, then a Ph.D. I became an English professor. So, my first husband was right, my intelligence would save me. I vowed in the year after her murder that I would never find myself in that position again. Neither my life nor my children's lives would ever be at the whim of some man every again. And I have held true to that promise.

Long gone is that rickety camper trailer. Long gone are the food stamps and welfare checks and standing in line waiting for free cheese. Long gone is that frightened teenage girl who was scared to hold her own baby and even more scared to admit it.

There is nothing I can do to bring my daughter back. I have accepted that, but it doesn't stop me from wishing, once a year, on her birthday that I could. There is a room here for her and one for her brother Nicholas. I hope that if I am ever blessed with another child that they won't mind sharing the space. Another child could never replace the ones that I have lost, but maybe, just maybe, holding a little one in my arms again, will ease the pain just a bit more.

I love you, Samantha Christine. Happy Birthday, my darling daughter.

Finding Hope

August 14, 2010 at 1:17 pm

LATELY, I HAVE BEEN having long talks with my friends about their teenaged children. All of them are having problems with their kids' behavior. Of course, my first reaction is that adolescence is horribly difficult to navigate and it is no wonder their teens are acting out. And, in typical me fashion, this made me think more about the teenaged me.

I have spoken of me as a young person here before. I was a troubled child and a wreck as a teen. I was Emo before Emo came to the Valley. I was withdrawn, sad, brooding. I wrote poetry, mostly dark, not to understand my anguish better but to represent it. "See, it hurts to be me."

In the past several years, I have spent a lot of time pondering that time in my life. In some ways, I was not a bad kid. I didn't use drugs. I didn't get arrested. No, I was bent on self-destruction, but at the time, I didn't see it that way. I had a very clear sense of right and wrong, and when I did something wrong, my wrong-o meter certainly chimed, which did make me stop for a moment. But most of the time I did whatever it was anyway.

I drank. I had sex. I ran away from home. So, what made me act out?

It would be easy to blame my parents. I mean, my home life was rocky to say the least. My parents were self-involved people who really had little idea about how to parent. Their own examples were troubling. Both of them came from abusive homes back when beating your kids with a razor straps was cool.

But it wasn't really the abuse at home that made me want to chase boys and smoke in the alley behind the skating rink. Rather, it was a combination of factors that ultimately lead up to a singular point: lack of hope.

And I blame this lack of hope not on my parents or their parents or my teen friends alone. Oh no, this lack of hope was embedded in me in my genetic material. The Ohio Valley (and the Mountain State itself) can be a hopeless place. Growing up here was stifling. I had no hopes, no dreams, no aspirations beyond tomorrow. I am not sure if it was better for middle class and upper middle class kids, but for poor kids like me, the next meal, the next morning, was really all there was to look forward to.

I know this may sound grim, but that was my mindset at the time. I could not imagine the point in getting good grades in school. After all, there was nothing after high school. College wasn't even a consideration. I never knew anyone who went besides my teachers, and surely, I could not be a teacher.

I loved writing, reading, cats, singing, science, history, basketball, and art. I entered competitions (like spelling bees) and won. But my parents had no interest at all in my schooling. I could have brought home straight Fs and my parents would have cared less. They were equally unimpressed with As. I am sure it has to do with their own personal philosophies of education. They both dropped out of school in the eighth grade. But those philosophies were rooted in the Valley mentality. In the 60s and 70s jobs were plentiful here, and no education, not even a high school diploma, was required.

Nonetheless, I absolutely loved learning. I could not get enough of new stuff! I even enrolled myself in summer school for gifted kids and spent part of my summers learning about the history of my state and astrology because I would rather be learning than doing anything else. I think that if one of my parents would have caught that spark, I would have had kept that focus.

Instead, I was sucked in by popular culture, which said that the value of a woman was her relationship to her man. The summer of my 13th year I read 12 paper grocery bags full of romance novels. I was reading four a day of these adult-themed books. In those pages I learned that women cared only about finding a man to spend her life with. First, he would resist her. Then, he would fall in love with her. Sometimes he would rape her, and then she would fall in love with him. WTF? This message was repeated to me on the big screen, too.

So, like most little girls, my first dream in life was to become a vet because I looooved kitties (still do!). Then, it was to become a lounge singer like Alice, who worked at Mel's Dinner and lounge sang at night at a local single's bar. But when the career aspirations dried up for lack of encouragement and hope, my singular focus became romantic love and getting out of my house. What I didn't realize then was that I had the power to get myself out. I did not need a boy to help me do that.

I am not dismissing the wonderfulness that is romantic love. I am married to the love of my life. But what I didn't understand then is that my happiness in life did not depend on being with a boy. It took me a very long time to figure that out. By then I had left a path of destruction around me far more sizable than the cartoon Tasmanian devil ever did. I hurt myself. I hurt others.

I guess what I am getting at here is that I do not think my situation was set in stone. I think that at any point along the way I could have been saved and if given the tools (hope) I could have even saved myself. Instead, I sought a way out, a way to be happy, through others, and low and behold, a co-dependent was born.

You must be wondering what could have been done for me to help me out back then. Well, I don't have all the answers and probably never will, but here is what I think:

1. Yelling at me and making more rules WOULD NOT have helped. In fact, more confinement made me act out even more.
2. Beating me did not help. I just ran away from home.
3. If an adult with good intentions and connections to academia or something beyond the trailer park would have

taken an interest in me and helped me see other possibilities, I might have found a way out.
4. If I would have developed my self-esteem, it would have made pursuing boys (and later men) a completely different experience. I know there is a lot of negative talk about teachers who work on building their young pupils' self-esteem, but I have seen it work in my own classroom. Telling a young person that he or she is creative, smart, inquisitive, or whatever true observation you can make can change that person's entire outlook on life.
5. If I would have had been role models in my age group, I think I would have been less likely to get involved in activities that harmed me. Not all of my friends went down the wrong road, but I had enough friends from troubled homes to hold my hand down the path of self-destruction.

All that said, I am who I am. There is no two ways about that. And part of who I am was developed in the crucible of those tender years where I was just discovered my Self. I have very few regrets of that time, but among my biggest is that I wish I would have treated other people more lovingly, but I am still learning how to do that.

Patting Myself on the Back

August 15, 2010

I HAVE ALWAYS been fascinated by what people who don't write do when they can't sleep. My Dad used to get up in the middle of the night and eat bread and butter sandwiches and drink glass after glass of milk. My grandma used to sit in the lights-out kitchen smoking, the red fiery dot of her cigarette the only clue to her presence. Me, I get up and I write.

Long before I ever owned a computer or even could construct a complete sentence, I would get up in the middle of the night, my head loaded with troubles, and write. Here it is 2 a.m. and I find myself restless with worry, not for myself but for someone I love. Given there is nothing I can do right now to help that person, I know I must turn my attention elsewhere or never get to sleep.

So, here I am writing.

Tonight's topic, which might be an undercurrent adding to my restlessness, is change. Not the kind you find in your pocket or in the dryer vent or in your couch cushions (always a bonus), but the kind a person undergoes within. Obviously, the way I and others have changed and continue to change is a main, but this recent spur of thought has to do with the recent reunion get together I attended the other day.

It was for the class ahead of me, but I went because so many people encouraged me to go. I had a great time, but this entry is not about what happened while I was at the event, but rather what happened before and after.

All the way up until I was in my car on the way to the location, I was fine. I was getting ready and listening to music and enjoying my afternoon. But as soon as I took the exit to my hometown, I panicked. I was suddenly nervous about walking in the door and seeing all of those people for the first time in 20 years. (Some of them I have seen more recently.) I wasn't so concerned I had second thoughts, but rather I had doubts about myself.

Every person doubts herself from time to time. I mean, I think we would not be very good people if we didn't question our motivations now and again. But in that moment, I felt 15 again. So, I did the only thing I knew to do: make a call.

I called one of my very best friends. I explained to him my feelings, and he immediately went into awesome friend mode, throwing compliments at me so fast I could barely catch them. It was just what I needed. I pulled into the parking lot of the pub and jumped out and walked right in.

On the drive back, though, I pondered that whole scene. I suppose most people would be nervous in a situation like that, but I think it was more than nerves of, "will they like me now," than, "do I like me now?" Have I really changed or have I pretended to change? Did I really change who I am? Or have I merely changed my friend group and zip code?

I mean, a person can completely reinvent herself by getting a new crowd of people to hang around with and moving to another city, but I wonder, if you didn't change, would you be able to hide your flaws forever?

So, I called my friend back, and he said something that made so much sense that I pulled over to write it down: "You are not who you were then. You are who you are now. And that is wonderful to me."

Perhaps, then, instead of worrying about whether I have really changed since high school, I should take my own advice and worry only about the now. I do like who I am today. I am always a work in progress, but it doesn't really matter if I have changed since then, but it matters if I can respect myself in the morning, so to speak. And, you know what, I can!

I am not perfect, but if part of who we are is reflected in the people who fill our lives, then I must be doing something right, because I have the best friends in the world.

A Few Words on Waiting

August 18, 2010

I AM PROBABLY one of the world's worst waiters. No, I don't mean I trip and spill your grilled trout in your lap at Red Lobster. I mean, I really stink at waiting for something to happen or not to happen.

I suppose it is just part of my identity as a must-have-now American, but I think it has more to do with my Type A personality. If

A Few Words on Waiting

something needs done, I do it and then it is done. It is when other people and conditions are involved that make it difficult for me to sit back and WAIT.

I have written about the 2ww here before. That time between ovulation and a period or a positive pregnancy test. I am right in the thick of that wait, and it is even worse this cycle because I have no idea when I ovulated. The freedom that comes with not taking my temps every morning sure seems like a burden when I get to Day 33 in my cycle with no period. I mean, I could be late, but who's to say? The only dependable thing about a menstrual cycle is the number of days in the luteal phase. It is just about the same give or take a day every single cycle. BUT in order to know when to expect a period it is necessary to know when ovulation occurred.

So, I might be late. I might not. I have had pretty crummy cramping for a few days, which is rare for me, but no spotting. However, unlike me just five months ago, I am not going to take a pregnancy test. I just cannot handle the heartache of another single line. Nope. Not gonna do that.

Instead, I am going to go to my doctor later today. It is a follow-up visit concerning the sonohystogram (the saline dye in the uterus test). He will go over those results and the results of my last round of blood work and give me the news. I feel so much like Sisyphus these days. I keep pushing this damn TTC boulder up the hill, and it rolls right back down again. The end result: no baby and a bigger doctor's bill.

If everything checks out as expected, I think he will recommend intrauterine insemination (IUI), which doesn't sound like too much fun. If that is the case, I am going to wait until Thanksgiving at the earliest to give it a shot. It requires some nasty drugs and many two-hour trips to and from his office, so I am going to need more time than this semester allows.

Hopefully, the news tomorrow will be good. As for the, "where is my period?" question... well, I just have to wait.

Doctor, Doctor, Give Me the News!

August 18, 2010

I ADMIT THE TITLE of this post is more than cheesy, but I am running out of doctor-themed titles, so there you go. I spent about three hours at the doctor's office today. Two hours waiting and one hour talking. In the end, the news is just what I expected and even a bit better.

He reviewed my bloodwork and said I have managed to beat PCOS into submission. He says I deserve a lot of credit for doing so. None of my levels, including my thyroid and insulin, are elevated. Better yet, my testosterone levels are normal and my ovarian reserve (egg count) is excellent. In other words, on paper I am pretty hot stuff.

All of my other tests show I am normal. Now, if you actually know me, you know that is a bit of a stretch. But my uterine cavity and remaining tube and all the other parts are in good working order. My chances are less some months because of the left tube being gone, but overall, I am in great shape.

One would think I would feel elated, and I do, especially about the PCOS butt kicking part, but I also feel aggravated. If I am a specimen of exquisite fertility, then why am I not pregnant?

He answered, "Well, there are some things we cannot explain."

I LMAOed, regrouped, and devise a working fertility plan:

Between Thanksgiving and New Year's, I will do a cycle of aggressive Clomid and IUI. Regular Clomid is pretty horrid. Aggressive Clomid will be super horrid. In addition to the plain old psychopath-producing, ovulation inducer that is Clomid, I will have to inject myself with hCG (the pregnancy hormone), which will make me ovulate. Then, they will inject me with my husband's very best sperm. Then, I will have to use progesterone suppositories for...three months! I have used those before, and I gotta say, they are pretty terrible. In any case, he is thinking that this just might work.

If it doesn't, then we might do another kind of IUI with full-force injectable hormones. If that doesn't work, then IVF next summer.

I don't like the sound of any of this. I am hoping somehow we manage to get the + sign on our own.

In any case, I will keep you all updated. It sure would be nice to get two pink lines this Saturday. It is our first wedding anniversary. But that might be asking too much.

Special Anniversary Edition

August 23, 2010

OVER THE PAST YEAR, I have dreamed of telling my husband I am pregnant. My first two pregnancies were unexpected and downright shocking, as was pregnancy #4 (blighted ovum). The only pregnancy that seemed to come along as planned was #3, but it turned out to be an ectopic, and it looked that way from the start. So, I have rarely been able to get excited about that first acknowledgement that a life is growing inside me.

We just celebrated our first wedding anniversary a few days ago. We spent four days of quality time together, and it was like a fairytale in some ways. So much time in each other's arms, wandering through a botanical garden, having dinner at our favorite restaurant, and kissing in the exact spot on the lake where we were married. I couldn't have dreamed up a more perfect weekend.

Feeling I might be on a roll, I took a pregnancy test on the morning of our anniversary. I mean, how much more terrific would it have been than to turn to my husband and say, "We are going to have a baby!"

Unfortunately, the test was negative. It made me feel sad for maybe 15 minutes, then I snuggled up with him on the couch and let it go. I wasn't about to let it spoil such a tender moment or any other part of our weekend together.

Being able to let go is a new practice and one that is becoming more effortless as time goes by. It required concentrated effort at first, but it has gotten easier.

And yet, it is not foolproof.

I still haven't started my period yet, but I know that it is about to arrive. I had that weird muscle spasm feeling last night and felt barfy this morning, so it won't be long now. Knowing this, I walked into a room of pregnant women with babies this morning.

First, a colleague announced that she was pregnant with her fourth child. (Her youngest is just six months old.) Then, a colleague wheeled in her newborn, who remained with us all day. I did pretty darn good for the most part. I mean, I focused on the task at hand, but those cranky, old voices started chattering:

- Why does she get to have four kids, and I don't get to have any?
- If all of my kids had lived, I would have four, too. (19, 9, 7, and 4)
- I should not have to listen to babies crying all day.
- I wish I was pregnant.
- I wish I had a baby.
- I wish I could just run out of this room and jump into the river and drown.

That went on off and on throughout the morning, but by lunchtime I was able to replace those thoughts with other thoughts, positive ones, and focus on the NOW.

And you know what? My period is probably going to start tomorrow morning, and I will be glad to see it come because then I will be on to the next cycle. But really, I will be glad to see it come because it proves that I am healthy and fertile...in my own way and that isn't all that bad!

Calgon, Take Me Away!

August 24, 2010

I GUESS THIS IS JUST a carryover from yesterday's pregnancy/baby drama or maybe it is PMS, but I am feeling sad. There is no better word, I guess. Melancholy, perhaps. Out of sorts, maybe. But sad seems most apt.

My husband has been out on the road for a couple of days, and I have been working hard, not sleeping well, and my period will be here in two days. All of these come together to make me feel so tried and sad.

I had a great day with my niece. It is always so flattering when people think she is my daughter. She is such a terrific young woman.

But now I am sitting alone at my desk preparing for the school year that arrives in just a few short days.

I am tired of thinking. I am tired of reading. I am tired.

I guess everyone is entitled to an evening of sad and blah every now and again. Perhaps a walk or some yoga will snap me out of my funk. Better yet, maybe I should just hang out with the sad for a while. Fighting emotions is not helpful, even though I have lived a great deal of my life doing just that. Maybe I'll take option 3, phone a friend.

The Big Reveal

August 25, 2010

I AM PREGNANT. Two weeks pregnant. Right this minute, I have a cute little ball of cells growing and dividing inside me. I hope it has red hair. LOL

I was momentarily (and I mean, like two minutes) hesitant about sharing the news so soon into the pregnancy. After all, anything can happen, and I have a history of pregnancy and infant loss.

However, I chose to disclose the great news just hours after I got the results because I knew you would want to know and because this is all part of my journey. No matter what happens in this pregnancy, it is important for me to be able to write about it here because I can tell you there are some long, nail-biting nights ahead.

How I found out that I am pregnant is a funny story, of course. I started thinking that this cycle was strange about a week ago when all cheeses smelled rancid to me. Then, last night I opened a package of brand new mozzarella and almost hurled. Still, I was sure I was just biding my time until my period came. I had the muscle spasm-like feelings in my uterus (I have those instead of cramps) and my breasts were sore. I kept checking for spotting...nothing.

So, I headed up to bed around 3 a.m. last night after working on some writing. I saw the last remaining pregnancy test on the counter (I tested on my anniversary four days ago), and took it. I mean, why not? Within seconds the test turned positive.

At first, I didn't believe it. I could buy a new Mac Book with the money I have spent on pregnancy tests over the years. But, sure enough within seconds that plus sign popped up and stayed there. I didn't have to squint to see it. I screamed (only the cats were here to hear me), "I'm pregnant!"

I immediately took my cup of pee (I prefer to dip than to pee on the stick), poured into a container with a lid, and decided to go to Walmart and buy more tests. I paused for a second to see if my late night friend (who is always in on my 3 a.m. drama) was online, and there she was! So glad to see her there. I told her the results and my plans to go buy more tests.

I drove to Walmart and bought three different brands of tests. I then raced back out to my car, and right there under the pole lights, I dipped those sticks in my butter bowl of pee. One after another after another they came out positive.

Now, you might think, wow, that is pretty gross (spilling it on myself was), but if you have ever wanted something so much, then you know the sort of rabid, nervous feeling that was going through me. I had to know for sure, and I had to know right then!

I drove home, all the way chanting, "I love you. I love you. I love you." to the little being building inside of me. I am scared, but I am going to try so hard to remain positive. I am sending love and light and warmth to this new life, the life I made with my husband.

By this time, it was 4 a.m. My friend was still online and we talked and talked and talked. I debated about when to call Jim with the news. He was sleeping in his truck in Virginia, so far away. Plus, I was afraid to tell him while he was on the road.

I held out until 6 a.m. when I knew he would be awake and called him. He was so incredibly thrilled! I could hear the smile in his voice!

As soon as I hung up, I called my doctor's office to schedule a blood test to confirm all of these HPTS.

Too tired to sleep, I read and talked to everyone who was awake. Just as I fell asleep around 8, the doctor's office called and sent me to the lab. Three hours later, they called to confirm: I am pregnant! My hCG level was 113, more than enough to confirm pregnancy.

It is still hard to believe. I can't quite come to grips with it. I think it will take a long while for it all to sink in. Just for a moment, I thought about all I have to give up over the next nine months: motorcycle rides with my husband, sushi, espresso, alcohol (not really a problem), sprouts, and all that I will have to go through, endless doctor's appointments, blood work, and exhaustion. But if that is ALL I have to do to have a healthy child, then it is no sweat. I can live without breve cappuccinos and salmon rolls.

I want to end this entry with a thank you! Thank you all so much for praying, hoping, wishing, and most of all, caring. I KNOW that your positive energy has helped me on this journey. I hope that you take as much joy in this moment as I do. I share it with you! (You'll all take turns babysitting, too, right? LOL). But don't stop reading, we have a long way to go from here.

And a Mama Lion Is Born

August 26, 2010

ANYONE WHO KNOWS ME knows I am pretty easygoing in many areas of my life. Healthcare is not one of them.

Given that it took me eight years to get diagnosed with Polycystic Ovarian Syndrome and shoddy (you know I wanted to write shitty, so I just did) pre-natal care cost me my son's life and almost my own, I don't trust doctors to always have my best interests at heart. I'm a pretty smart broad, and I can read medical journals and get the jargon. I have made the choice to be my own advocate. If I am willing to fight for myself, you better believe I will come out swinging for my lion cub.

At my reproductive endocrinologist's office in Cincinnati, they would monitor a pregnancy for the first eight weeks, and then turn the patient over to an OB/GYN. The idea was they could monitor a woman very closely for the first two months (after the heart beat is confirmed) in order to track the pregnancy. In fact, they caught my ectopic back in 2004, long before it could ever be visualized on ultrasound. They did so by monitoring the level of hCG (the pregnancy hormone) in my blood. It became obvious after a week or so I was pregnant with an ectopic because my hCG numbers did not double as they should, but rather climbed (4,000) and fell (2) rapidly and unexpectedly. The ectopic was never visualized on ultrasound, but if not for their vigilance, my health and life would have been in jeopardy.

OB/GYNs do not monitor most pregnant women that closely. By the end of the first six weeks, I had eight ultrasounds. The same is true for the blighted ovum I had in 2006. If she hadn't been following that pregnancy closely on ultrasound, there is no way we would have known that the yolk sack was empty. And later, she had to do a D&C, because I did not miscarry completely on my own.

All of that said, I am considered high risk, and I wanted to be treated like I am high risk, which means more early monitoring and intervention if necessary.

So, I spent the day on the phone with doctor's offices. It was annoying and stressful. The earliest anyone would see me is September 14.

You might say, "Gee, that is not so far off."

To me, it is. After the fourth call, I decided to go right to the source: Maternal and Fetal Medicine at Magee. I go to Magee for fertility care, and this just seems like the best choice. They will consider me high risk when I walk in the door, and they are experts at dealing with all kinds of complicated pregnancies.

Best yet, I scored an appointment for September 7. I can live with that, especially since I know they will do a great job. In addition to excellent care, they provide hospital-to-hospital care, which means if I have a problem in my hometown, they will send someone to pick me up and take me to Magee. In addition, they have a 24-hour help line and 24-hour service. I'm in.

Perhaps some of you will think I am being extreme, but my health and the baby's health are important to me, and I will do whatever I can to bring a healthy baby home. Even if it means I have to hire and fire four doctors in one day!

Our First Day Back in the Classroom

August 29, 2010

THE CUB AND I head back to school tomorrow. I have 145 students ready to be taught a little something about writing. I am excited to head back but worried about the physical challenges of teaching five classes, the most I have taught in my 15-year career.

I have a couple of breaks throughout the day, but it is a long day (6:30 a.m.-5:00 p.m.) with a lot of walking (about 5 miles). My plan is to stay hydrated and fed. Drinking and snacking all day should keep my blood sugar and energy stable.

I am feeling less worried about the success of this pregnancy as each day goes by, but I still freak out just a little when I go to the bathroom, so afraid to see spotting. But so far, we have made it to 4 weeks and 6 days. I have mild cramping on and off, which is normal. Of course, my breasts feel like someone beat them with a hammer, I have to pee all the time, and I have pretty severe nausea in the morning. (I have never had morning sickness.) All of those are good signs that my body is making plenty of progesterone to sustain the embryo until the placenta is formed.

Right now, the cub is really small, the size of an apple seed, but he or she sure seems big to me. Big in my heart!

First OB/GYN appointment in nine days.

Annoying Paranoia

August 30, 2010

WE MADE IT THROUGH the first day back. It was a long day, but I kept hydrated and fed just like I needed to, and everything seemed to go okay. Of course, I was tired by the end of the day, but I have a lively 3 p.m. class, so that should keep me going until I head out at 4. It is only three days a week, and I am thankful for that.

Despite the busyness of the day, I still could not shut off the worry track in the back of my head. Since I can't help but share my inner monologues here....

> *Why are my breasts no longer sore? I have only peed four times this morning, is that enough? Was that a cramp? No, wait, it was more like a twinge. No, seemed like a cramp. Oh, just some gas. My abdomen is huge. Do I look like Violet Beauregarde, just in black pants? My throat feels sore. Am I coming down with the flu? Should I hold my breath going through this tunnel? That is definitely a sore throat.*

I annoy myself! It's a good thing the cub can't hear my thoughts. I am sure he or she would be driven insane and start begging to get out by Thanksgiving.

All the while, I have no reason at all to think there is anything wrong with this pregnancy. I have some strikes against me (over 35, PCOS, obesity, previous pregnancy losses, conceived late in my cycle, husband over age 40, etc.), but as far as the pregnancy itself, it seems fine.

I guess the only way I will be able to calm down is when I reach each milestone. Here are some big ones I am aiming for:

- The first Doctor's appointment (Sept. 7)
- Seeing the heartbeat on transvaginal ultrasound (week 6+, hopefully, Sept. 7)
- Hearing the baby's heartbeat for the first time (week 12+)
- Week 13 (we'll be out of the first trimester, which decreases our loss rate tremendously)
- Week 26 (two weeks after my son, Nicholas, was born)
- Week 32 (a very good chance if born premature, the baby will be developed enough and just fine)
- week 36 (a live healthy birth)
- age 70 (the "baby" will be in his or her 30s, and I won't have to worry too much; lol)

Two-Week Wait

I know some of you must think I am crazy, and I suppose I am to a point. But, I am living in the shadow of loss, and it takes extra effort to push the sunlight through.

Every night before I go to sleep and throughout the day, I send happy thoughts and love to the little cub. I am not anxious in the sense that I am nervous. More like, I am concerned, but I have to say, it is getting old.

September 2010

Scared to Look

September 6, 2010 at 7:12 pm

THE HUSBAND, the cub, and I spent a very nice weekend in the mountains of our home state. It really is an amazing place, and now that we have our own little camping area that we found on our last trip, it makes it all the more special, like going home. For the most part, the trip was quite enjoyable, but I could not stop worrying about the cub completely.

It was cold at night, but we kept warm snuggled in our packs, zipped together. We went for short walks, nothing too strenuous, and spent a lot of time talking about how much we loved spending time alone, especially in the woods. We met many interesting people, including a woman who had just had a baby about six weeks ago after trying for a year to get pregnant. (She was only 22, and her son, Orion, was lovely.)

Perhaps the most interesting part of the trip was when Jim and I visited the place where he used to camp as a boy. It was along the Dry Fork River and was absolutely stunning. He remembered that there was an island near his camp where a woman lived in a one-room house. We not only found the island and the woman, but we discovered that her house had become something! She has spent the last 30 years building it into an absolute oasis, complete with river rock gardens, a lookout tower with a spiral staircase, and incredible, carved woodworking that is beyond description. She very happily showed us her handiwork, and we both fell in love with the place and her artistic talents.

When we originally approached her, Jim said, "I want to show my wife where I spent some of the happiest days of my childhood." It was touching, and we both agreed that we want to build something spectacular like that together some day.

We also took in a great show at the local coffee house/hippie eatery and an art gallery opening. (Love me some granola mountain folk.) Both of us felt swallowed up by the glow of the pregnancy. He kept saying, "Married just a year and a wonderful baby on the way." It seemed that every step I took, I felt renewed in the sense that I was creating a life, right then, right there.

But in the back of my mind, I still carried concern. Was that a twinge? Was that a cramp? Ouch. That seems like one-sided pain. Yes, it is one-sided pain. (And it was, but I am convinced it was from the long ride. Even though we got out and walked every 45 minutes or so, it was a lot of sitting cramped up.)

I have had mild cramping off and on since before I found out I was pregnant. It comes and goes and never really worried me because I wasn't spotting blood, until this morning.

After a lovely night of coziness with the husband, all clean and fresh in our own bed, I woke up to very faint pink spotting. Every time thereafter, though, the spotting was gone. We spent the rest of the day enjoying a few more hours of each other's company, including looking at baby cribs, something I thought we wouldn't do until seven months, or at least until we were more clearly out of danger.

The spotting came back about three hours later, and is still there. It is now brown.

I know for a fact that spotting after intercourse during pregnancy is normal. I know it because I have read it, I have had other women tell me that, and I have had a doctor tell me that. And yet, I am scared out of my mind. The thought of finally getting pregnant and then losing the baby is just hard to accept.

And so I won't accept it.

There is no good reason to accept it. I go in tomorrow for my first appointment. I will demand an ultrasound if one is not offered to me. I will ask them to measure my hcg and progesterone levels. I will know one way or another the status of this pregnancy when I leave there tomorrow afternoon.

Until then, I will continue to repeat the mantra: I am pregnant and the baby is healthy. Please, say it with me.

Repeat After Me

September 7, 2010 at 8:20 am

JUST FOUR MORE HOURS and I should know if this pregnancy is viable or not. After spotting yesterday, I woke up this morning with low cramping. I have high hopes that all is well and this is just a hormonal response, but I won't know much of anything until I get that ultrasound done. Even that might be inconclusive.

I recall the dreaded blighted ovum, a pregnancy/miscarriage that went on for MONTHS! From March through May, I continued to see my doctor. One day it was a missed abortion (missed miscarriage), the next time it was a viable pregnancy, and on and on and on. My ex-husband was so frustrated with the process that he felt it should be called WTF?! Eventually, the pregnancy/miscarriage ended in a D&C.

I go back and forth from thinking things are fine to thinking they are not, dreading the phone call to my husband this afternoon if I have bad news. It is a one hour drive to the doctor's office. I will repeat and keep repeating: I am pregnant and the baby is healthy all the way up until I get the ultrasound.

Keep us in your thoughts, prayers, meditations. The cub and I will be fine!

First Ultrasound

September 7, 2010 at 2:40 pm

I HAD MY FIRST ultrasound today. The good news is that they found a gestational sac in my uterus, which means no ectopic. The less-than-confirming news is that there was nothing in it, no yolk sack or anything. I am worried that this is a blighted ovum again, but she said there is no way we can say that at all. She was not worried. She says things are not out of the ordinary and everything seems fine.

The machine dated the gestational sac at 5w5d. My software, using my guessed at O date, says I am 6w1d. So much can happen in such a short time.

I have a follow up u/s scheduled for one week from now. She said if we don't see a yolk sac then, we have trouble.

She also confirmed that spotting after sex is totally normal.

So, for the rest of this week, I am going to walk this Earth like I am any other pregnant woman. I cannot control what happens in this pregnant, but I can control how I feel about it. I love my little cub and will keep sending it sweet thoughts.

Rough Day

September 8, 2010 at 7:50 pm

I HAD A ROUGH DAY today. I didn't sleep well last night, and I had to get up at 5 am to take my husband to work. I headed off to work myself at 7:15 and didn't get home until 5 pm. The day itself, however, was filled with anxiety, a sugar crash, and absolute exhaustion.

I had an absolutely great morning. No spotting. No cramps. Sunshine. High energy. Wonderful!

By Noon, however, things were not going so well. I was starting to feel light headed, my hands started shaking, and I couldn't think clearly. I assumed that I just hadn't eaten enough, so I had the ONLY thing within reach: an Orange Crush. (Yeah, it was sooo tasty. I hadn't had one in many, many years.) Anyway, halfway through the bottle, I was back to my normal self.

I taught three more classes, found spotting (brown/pink), and walked back to my car. I barely made it there. I honestly thought that I was going to have to sit down on the sidewalk. I could barely function. I started thinking...migraine! Yes, indeed a big migraine was coming. Unfortunately, I also experienced a panic attack along with it.

I have an hour drive to get home. I called Jim as soon as I could. He did his best to calm me and convince me that I was not having a stroke or a heart attack. But I was so anxious, all I could think about was the basalar (sometimes called vascular) migraine I had in 2008. It was eerily similar: complete exhaustion, garbled thinking, difficulty speaking clearly, and visual disturbances. Thankfully, I did not lose my vision like last time. The last time I lost half of my vision. So incredibly scary.

I am feeling much better now, but what remains is the headache itself. It is painful, and I feel like I have a hangover. I came home and immediately crashed on the couch.

The good news is that the minor spotting from earlier today is gone completely. No cramps either.

Hopefully, baby is okay.

Meanwhile, given that the last headache was caused by exhaustion, I plan on combatting future problems by eating much more throughout the day (I have been eating six small meals, but I think I need a couple of bigger ones), calling off work if I have had too little sleep, taking a very short nap at lunch time (15 minutes), and talking to my migraine guy about pregnancy-safe drugs.

Thankfully, I got home okay. It was a white-knuckle drive. I figured, though, that since you are all looking out for me that I would be just fine. Thanks!!

And Still...

September 10, 2010 at 6:51 pm

IT HAS BEEN a long week. It began with the end of a lovely weekend and ends with exhaustion, off-and-on brown spotting and mild anxiety.

The spotting began after sex on Monday morning and has continued through an ultrasound. Although it is nowhere near as heavy as it was on Tuesday morning, it is still there every fourth or fifth time I go to the bathroom. It makes me feel like I am going crazy. One minute I am fully certain that all is and will be well. Then, an hour or two later, I see the little spot on the tissue and I am back to being anxious. I am getting better at letting it go faster, but it is scary.

I want to have this child so badly that the mere thought of losing it is unbearable. At the same time, I acknowledge that most miscarriages happen for a reason, and I would not want to keep a little soul here on this Earth that is not capable of being. The most common reason for early miscarriage is genetic malformations in the embryo. If it needs to go, it needs to go.

But something in me just doesn't believe that this little cub is meant for anywhere else but in my arms. One of my Due Date Buddies from my online support group was told a week ago that she was would miscarry. She hasn't yet, and each day that she remains pregnant, she wakes up, hugs her abdomen, and says a solemn thank you for being able to carry the life just one more day.

I haven't been told anything of the sort, and other than the spotting, which does seem to have a non-uterine source, everything seems fine to me. I have pregnancy symptoms, including wretched tiredness, breast tenderness, mild cramping, bloating, nausea, and migraine!

If you have read my blog long enough, you know how difficult it is for me to let go. I know there is absolutely nothing I can do to change what happens here—either way. But I'll be damned if I wouldn't do something if I could.

I look around me and wonder how all of us ever got here, many of us quite normally. Creating a life is hard, frightening work. If desire and love alone were enough to produce a healthy child, I would be holding one in my arms as I type this. Instead, I wait, trying to distract myself. Trying not to panic when I see that one little dot of brown blood.

If you are praying and wishing for me and the cub, then send us waves of peace. Meanwhile, I will listen for his or her little roar. I know, I know, I know if the cub is anything like me or Jim, then he or she has a will of iron, which might be just what we need right now, but will make the teenage years unbearable.

A Wild Ride

September 11, 2010 at 10:09 pm

TODAY BEGAN FINE. Woke up cozy next to the husband. The house was chilly, but in a fall-is-here kind of way. We had tea and chatted. I was still spotting just a little, but it seemed to be clearing up. Then, my brother and his pregnant girlfriend stopped by, and she commented on my pregnancy glow, which to me just seems like a lot of acne. Not minutes after they left, a trip to the bathroom revealed heavier spotting, and I nearly threw up. In my mind, all I could see is that it is over.

The spotting never turned red, and I never had cramps with it, but it was pinker and heavier than it had been. I called my doctor, and he said go to the local ER. Jim drove me there, holding my hand all the way. Four hours later, we walked out with smiles on our faces that I could never have predicted and wouldn't have believed if the Oracle of Delphi put it forth!

We learned during our trials today.....

- that there is a yolk sac and a little person
- The Cub has a heartbeat: 113! Perfect!
- I got to hear the heartbeat, still very faint
- the pregnancy has progressed right on track to 6 weeks 2 days
- my cervix is closed and high
- there is no blood around my cervix or in my vagina, just brown gunk (leftover from the bleed)
- my hcg levels are 42,000 (which is just perfect)

The only negative thing we learned is that I have a cyst on my right ovary, which are common in pregnancy. I hope to learn more about that on Tuesday at my appointment with my ob.

All this means that everything is fine. The Cub is tucked away safely inside my uterus. In fact, she said that he or she is burrowed right into the middle of my back wall, which means less of a chance of developing a previa, like I did with Nicholas.

According to the American Pregnancy Association and other reliable sources, the pregnancy is 70-90% likely to remain viable!

To confirm and then re-confirm this fact over and over again in my mind and heart, I found a lovely necklace at Sak's while we were searching the mall for baby cribs (just to get an idea of price and style). I don't have my camera handy, so I will have to post tomorrow. Basically, the necklace is gold with four circles of various sizes. To me, they represent health and fertility. Every time I touch them, I will be reminded that as long as I am not bleeding red or doubled over with cramps, the Cub is fine and will be fine. I'm going to have a baby!

Cub Report

September 14, 2010 at 7:46 pm

KEEPING IT BRIEF tonight, since the Cub and I need our rest. Long day tomorrow.

We had our third ultrasound today, and everything looked great. Heartbeat: 130. Pregnancy measuring at 6w 4d. We are right on track.

Best yet, my doctors confirmed that my pregnancy is normal, and although they will continue to follow me closely (my next appt is not for another two weeks), I am free to enjoy life like any other pregnant gal. I am going to head back to the pool this weekend. I am so relieved.

Next milestone: week 14. We need to find out where the placenta implants. Hopefully, far far away from my cervix.

Now that I can relax a little, I plan on writing about issues other than Cub making....at least for the next few weeks.

You know what burns my biscuits?

September 15, 2010 at 5:59 pm

JUST WHEN I THOUGHT I was totally fine, I woke up at 3:30 am to severe right-sided pain: ovarian cyst rupture. Thankfully, I knew right away what was going on. "Luckily" I had had a cyst or two rupture in the past, but that didn't stop me from thinking, "Really? My spotting stops and now this?"

I could barely make it to my car to drive to work but by the time I got there, I was feeling a little better. The pain was almost entirely gone by the middle of the day.

I called my doctor just to be on the safe side and to report the situation. He said to take Tylenol. I decided to just deal with it. Don't want the Cub all drugged up.

Finally made it home, but not before bursting into tears over dinner with hubby. It was a long day, he was in a grumpy mood, and I just needed to take a nap. And that is just what I am doing. The cats and I are cozy on the sofa. We have our blanket and herbal tea. Working from home tomorrow. Sounds like a pajama day for me and the Cub.

The Cub's Debut

September 16, 2010 at 8:32 am

THE CUB IS ABOUT the size of an apple seed with a tadpole appearance. Cutest human in the world, but I could be biased.

A Word (or Two) about GAD

September 16, 2010

YOU KNOW I HAVE some trouble with anxiety. Although many of you have recommended I just relax or go with it (good advice, by the way), for someone with generalized anxiety disorder (GAD), it is not that easy.

I have probably had GAD since childhood, but it really did not manifest itself until after my daughter was murdered in 1991. I suffered from post-traumatic stress, which worsened my anxiety. My mental state for years following her death was precarious. My threshold for having an anxiety attack was quite low, and something as simple as a loud noise or even a pleasant surprise would make my hands shake and heart beat fast.

I suffered bouts of anxiety in the years that followed, especially during my pregnancy with my son and after his death. Two weeks

A Word (or Two) about GAD

after he died, I was scheduled to get my gallbladder removed, and I ended up freaking out right outside the operating room. I ripped the IV out of my arm and ran through the halls, bare butt hanging out the back of my ill-fitting gown. I had to get out of there. (Yeah, it is funny to me now, too.)

You see, anxiety disorder is not simply worrying. Everybody worries. The difference is that anxiety can be incapacitating, especially if it turns to panic, which is what happened to me in 2003. I had been taking Clomid to try to conceive a child. As I have mentioned here, Clomid makes most women crazy.

It made me have panic attacks. I remember more than once not being able to get in the shower because I was afraid of inhaling hot steam and aspirating. (It's not logical, but that is the nature of the illness.) I missed many days of work that year because I literally could not leave. I could not walk out the front door and even think about teaching a class.

To give you a better idea of what I was going through, here is a list of my symptoms:

- Rapid heart rate
- Sweating
- Trembling
- Shortness of breath
- Hyperventilation
- Feeling like I am going to die
- Abdominal cramping
- Chest pain
- Dizziness
- Faintness
- Tightness in my throat
- Trouble swallowing

One of the worst things about panic attacks is the intense fear you'll have another panic attack. If you have had four or more panic attacks and have spent a month or more in constant fear of another attack, you may have a condition called panic disorder, a type of chronic anxiety disorder.

With panic disorder, you may fear having a panic attack so much that you avoid situations where they may occur. You may even be unable to leave your home (agoraphobia), because no place feels safe.

Eventually, I figured out what was going on with me, and I sought help, but it took me a long time to find any. In the meantime, I attempted to medicate myself with alcohol, milk, food, and anything at all. I became desperate. At one point, I was having two panic attacks per day!

I finally found a doctor who would treat me. He gave me buspirone, which I took daily. I took the lowest dose possible. It began to help. Then, I read every single book I could find about anxiety disorder. The book that helped me the most was the *Anxiety and Depression Workbook*. It taught me that even though there is often no apparent reason for a panic attack, there are some factors that are known to set them off:

- caffeine
- salt
- processed foods
- MSG
- artificial sweeteners
- foods high in sugar
- lack of sleep

I developed my own plan for beating anxiety. Along with the medication, I starting keep a mood journal and came up with strategies that worked for me. In addition to changing my diet, I added more exercise to my routine, I made sure I got enough sleep, I cut down on my caffeine intake, and I stopped watching or reading things that upset me (shows like ER and other medical dramas, for example).

I also learned techniques for getting through panic attacks. Sometimes I would splash cold water in my face or I would wear a rubber band and snap it when I felt it starting. I would also hold my breath or take deep breaths until it passed. Riding out the anxiety was better than fighting it. The panic would go away within half an hour, but it was hell on Earth getting through that seemingly short period of time.

It took me three years, but I managed to stop having full-blown panic attacks, and I reduced my overall anxiety tremendously. I will never be cured of GAD, but I can live with it. Last week, I had my first panic attack in more than a year. It was so unfamiliar to me I had forgotten the hallmarks. I honestly felt like I was dying. Once I realized it was panic, I breathed deeply and rode it out. I emerged shaky and irritated, but I was okay.

I guess this post has a couple of purposes:

1. To educate all of you about anxiety disorder (I hope you don't already know about it from personal experience) and
2. To explain why sometimes I probably seem a little overwrought about situations that you might find easy to cope with.

In dealing with anxiety, knowledge is power. Unfortunately, I wish that I could have remained ignorant about this horrifying disorder, but it is now a devil that I know.

Mind Over Matter

September 20, 2010

AROUND NOON TODAY, I felt this sharp stabbing pain in my pubic bone. It lasted for just about a second. It scared me, though, because it was severe. I went off to class and tried to forget about it, but I started feeling crampy. Once I became distracted by teaching, the cramping magically disappeared. Now, it has returned.

I KNOW that cramping in pregnancy is normal. This, by the way, is not doubled-over cramping, but more of a fluttery feeling that I get right before I start my period. I am one of the lucky women who does not get cramps more than once a year, at most, during a period, so that is why these fluttering, spasmodic feelings are frightening.

And...

I posted a question about my stabbing pubic bone pain to my online support group. The only response to my query: "I experienced the exact same pain one week before I miscarried." Guess what? The stabbing pain and crampy fluttering has returned.

I truly believe that most of the sensation is in my head, but like with other parts of anxiety disorder, I am unable to convince myself that is true. Even if the pain is real (or realer than the exaggerated feedback I am receiving), there is no reason to believe it is significant. What's remarkable is I had horrendous pain with the cyst rupture last week and yet I didn't panic. In fact, I drove to work and taught all day.

I guess because this pain earlier today was a brand new sensation it has me spooked. I have clutched my talisman so many times today I nearly choked myself.

Given that I am alone tonight once again, I am going to go upstairs and take a warm (but not hot) bath, read a book (actually, I am re-reading Joan Didion's *Slouching Toward Bethlehem*), and meditate cozy in my bed. What will be, will be. All I can do is respond. I am hoping it is just gas.

Energy Exchange Urgently Needed

September 21, 2010

EARLIER THIS EVENING my sister-in-law was rushed to a Pittsburgh hospital. She has pre-eclampsia and is only 29 weeks pregnant. The baby is not doing well. He is measuring two weeks behind.

They are doing what they can for her, including giving her magnesium and steroids. If they cannot stabilize her, they will have to take the baby. He is obviously very early.

If you have been praying for me and the Cub or sending us positive energy, please send all of it their way. They need it desperately right now.

I have been exactly where they are. My son did not live. I am hoping and praying that their son does. They are in far better hands than I was, so if modern medicine is the answer, let it be so.

My Nephew Is Here!

September 22, 2010

AT AROUND 4 AM, my nephew, Dylan, was born. The doctors said he was in good shape for being born so early (29 weeks) and that he can breathe on his own. He will be in NICU for about two months as long as he progresses as expected. I have seen his picture, and he is quite handsome.

I am heading up to see him and my family in the next hour or so. It will be difficult. The last time I was in NICU, *my son* was in the incubator, but he was dying. I am absolutely grateful for the great prognosis my nephew has been given, so perhaps the images of those sad, sad days almost ten years ago will be overwritten by a preemie thriving.

I have a new nephew, which is just wonderful!

Thank you for sending me your thoughts and prayers. Updates to come.

Out, Damn'd Spot!

September 22, 2010

THOSE OF YOU LIT LOVERS had to know that I would eventually post an entry with this title. Given that I would not want to let you down, the Macbethian title appears at last. Of course, Lady M. was dealing with guilt there, and I, well, I am dealing with a whole different set of emotions.

I slept very little last night. My brother kept in constant communication with me (and I would have it no other way) as they made the agonizing decision to bring his son into the world two months early. In the end, it was all they could do to save Mom and baby. And so at around 4 a.m. my nephew Dylan came along.

I slept for a few hours, then drove the hour and 15 minutes to the hospital. It was a precarious journey. It is located in a part of town with which I am unfamiliar, so I ended up getting lost four of five times before finally pulling into the parking garage. (My GPS, by the way, lead me astray. Thank you, TomTom!)

Once I got the hospital, it took me 45 minutes to find my sister-in-law's room. The hospital, like just about every road into, out of, or in the middle of Pittsburgh, was under construction. Finally, I found my family. Mama was tired and frustrated because she hadn't been able to see her baby for more than a few minutes (both are hooked up to necessary machines), my brother was sleeping in a heap in the corner, and my Mom was looking frazzled but fine as she sat nearby waiting to lend a hand.

After lunch I was finally on my way to see Dylan. I was a little anxious as my brother and I entered the NICU and scrubbed up. So much of the routine was so familiar. The soap smelled the same. The incubators looked the same, even the baby quilts used to make the preemies cozy were reminiscent of the time my son Nicholas spent in the NICU.

But I reminded myself that I was not there to see a baby who was failing as it was so obvious that my son was from the start. (His odds of surviving the flight to Children's Hospital were 20%). Instead, I was here to see a baby that was given 90-95% odds. A baby who was born pink with a closed circulatory system and lungs that could breathe for him. I was going to see my nephew who would one day hound me (as his big brother is now) for money to take his date to Homecoming.

I followed my brother through a room of super small humans and leaned over his shoulder to catch my first glimpse of my own flesh and blood.

He took my breath away. So tiny and pink and just absolutely wonderful! He looked so healthy. He was not on a respirator. His machines did not continuously beep and ring like Nicholas' did. No. Not this baby. He is a perfect little person who just needs time to grow. We told him we loved him and said our goodbyes filled with hope that the next two months will pass by uneventfully, and Dylan will come home in time for Thanksgiving.

Yes, oh yes, being there, seeing him, made me miss my son in a way that nothing else would, but being with my nephew was worth any amount of grief.

On the way back to see his mama, I stopped at the restroom and discovered that I was spotting again. Seeing that clump of brown on the tissue, I immediately mumbled, "Fuck." Disgusted, angry, sad, and any negative emotion you can dream up, I walked back to the room with my brother. Of course, I couldn't tell my family. They had enough worries, so I got in my car and made my way slowly home.

In the nearly two hours of bumper-to-bumper traffic, I resolved not to worry about it. I KNOW that there is nothing that can be done to prevent a miscarriage this early. My doctor told me that more than once. So, I just drove (lurched) on. In fact, I was so not worried about it that I drove right by my doctor's office, when just a week ago, I would have stopped and begged to see someone. I was holding it together.

Then, the storm hit.

I finally got a break in traffic just outside the Fort Pitt Tunnel. Three lanes of people going 55, barreling for home. Just as I hit the crest of the first hill, the sky opened up and visibility shrank to zero. With my wipers at full speed, I could see nothing outside my car. A sheet of rain coated my windshield. It did not lessen.

Right there on 376 North, I finally lost it.

I was stuck in the left lane next to a Jersey barrier in blinding rain during rush hour traffic. I was spotting. My nephew was in NICU. And damn it, I felt so alone. I turned on my hazard lights and crept along, feeling my way blindly in the rain. There was no way to get over, or I would have sought the berm immediately. Instead, I cried.

I cried, and I cried, and I cried. I was alone. No one could help me. The Cub and I had only my Fusion for protection against potential out-of-control semis, flying road construction signs (there were many), and downed trees.

Miles and miles later, just a hundred feet before the West Virginia line (Oh beloved! My beloved!), the sun came out bright and furious. I rolled down my windows, wiped my eyes, and cranked Stone Temple Pilots the last several exits to home. Home. Home. Home.

We are alone, still, the Cub and I. But we are home at last, enjoying the comforts of our favorite chair, snugging with the kitties, and rejoicing in the knowledge that right at this moment all is well as far as we know. My nephew is in good hands, my spotting has stopped, and we are home. I think it is time for a nap. The Cub and I have had a long day.

I'm Still Here

September 26, 2010

It's been about four days since I made my harrowing post about my travels back from seeing my nephew in NICU. I have tried posting several times, but my workload has just gotten the better of me.

I have an appointment on Tuesday. I will get to see the baby again. I will post afterwards with an update. I promise!

Tomorrow and Tomorrow and Tomorrow

September 27, 2010

... really doesn't creep in this petty pace from day to day no matter what Willy S. had to say. There's nothing petty about any day. After all, it is all we got.

Sorry to wax philosophically here (I am in an 80s kind of mood), but I go in for my fourth ultrasound tomorrow, and I am a little nervous. One of three things could happen tomorrow:

- I see the Cub and everything is awesome.
- I see the Cub and things aren't going well.
- The Cub has died.

Now, I am not about to dwell on #3 there. Heck, I think I might as well kick #2 to the curb as well. Instead, I am going to watch the screen and see a little Cub measuring right along as expected. I am going to hear that little Cub's roaring heartbeat, too.

I have been worried the past few days that something is wrong because many of my pregnancy symptoms have faded or are gone entirely, but I have learned through my online support group that this is all normal. I am thankful that I am not horribly ill with morning sickness. I do have pretty severe mood swings, tiredness, headaches, acne, etc.

In other news, I will get to see my nephew, Dylan, tomorrow after my doctor's appointment. Getting to see two lovely babies in one day is surely a blessing.

I know you are wishing me luck tomorrow, and the Cub and I appreciate it. I promise to post an entry and a new Cub pic as soon as I can. Meanwhile, I will try my hardest not to let doubt creep in ... petty pace or not.

Me, My Cub, and I

September 28, 2010

I LEFT THIS HOUSE nearly 12 hours ago after a frantic phone call from my brother. A routine scan revealed bleeding on his son Dylan's brain. He was crying. I had to go.

The neurologist said that the bleeding was not life threatening, but would cause physical disability later in Dylan's life. They could not predict the extent or even the type, but they are 80% sure that he would not escape without some type of permanent problem. They are confident about his prognosis, though. He is no longer on oxygen, and he is eating well.

Around noon, they said I could hold him, but I am just not there yet. Just being in the room with all the incubators is still difficult for me. Those monitor sounds are frightening reminders of that agonizing week I spent with my son. But I so loved being able to visit with Dylan and tell him that I love him and that he will come home soon. The best part was hearing his little voice cry out while he was getting his diaper changed. I was still under heavy sedation when Nicholas was born, so I did not get to hear his one and only cry. His father described as a "soft wail." (He had a way with words.)

I left with my family around 2 and headed across town to my appointment.

My doctors are marvelous. They truly are the best doctors I have ever had. They spent two hours answering every single possible question I could have, doing an ultrasound and some other tests, and just making me feel comfortable with everything.

And now for the news you have all been waiting for:

I saw the Cub again, and s/he is doing absolutely great. S/he measured at 9 weeks (a bit ahead of schedule) with a heart rate of 186 b.p.m. which is just perfect. (At 9 weeks, the heart rate should be between 160 and 195 b.p.m.) I listened and listened to that lovely heartbeat hammering around inside me. I so wish I could have recorded it, so that I could listen to it every night before bed. (They sell home Doppler's , but I think it would make me insane.)

As I was leaving, my doctors told me I was now considered low risk!! In fact, one of my doctors said I am "the lowest risk patient in the practice." Hooray! I never thought I would hear that. My next appointment is a month away. A whole month! It will be hard to go that long without seeing the Cub, but I will get through it. I am going to try to schedule it for the day after my birthday. Such a good present!

Our next step is to go in for first trimester genetic screening. My odds of having a child with Down's syndrome are roughly 1 in 200. Screening at 10-12 weeks will be able to give me more specific odds. I think I would hold off on this until 20 weeks when they do a full body scan of the baby, but Jim wants to do the genetic screening sooner rather than later. I am okay with that and will set up an appointment tomorrow. I am fairly confident things will be fine, too.

I cannot explain how relieved I felt to see that heartbeat flashing away on the screen. After the scare with Dylan, getting good news about the Cub was just what I needed. Now, I plan to enjoy the next month until I see how big the Cub has grown. We're having a baby!

Screenings

September 30, 2010

I FINALLY FEEL like the Cub and I are "out of the woods" in terms of early miscarriage. Although anything can happen, the chances seem much less now we have seen the baby dating at 9 weeks. Since the ultrasound on Tuesday, I have felt freer and more comfortable being pregnant. My next appointment is scheduled right before my birthday. Unfortunately, now is the time to consider screening for birth defects.

I am lucky enough to be a patient at a world class hospital, which means the latest technology and procedures are available to me and the Cub. Between 11 and 13 weeks, pregnant women are eligible for something called a nuchal screening test, which I knew nothing about until my doctor mentioned it to me at my last appointment. In previous pregnancies, I was aware of amniocentesis, but this new test is done in the first trimester and amnio is done around 16 weeks. Like amnio, the nuchal scan/test will reveal the odds of the Cub having a genetic abnormality like Down's Syndrome or a neural tube defect.

The nuchal test (NT) looks at several pieces of the maternal/baby picture: maternal age, family history of genetic diseases, level of hCG (the "pregnancy hormone"), PPA, and the nuchal fold (a flap of skin on the back of the baby's head). The test is not invasive. They draw blood from me and ultrasound the Cub. The results will indicate the probability of whether or not the Cub will have a serious genetic disorder. I will get the results that day. If they are unfavorable, they will take a villi, or little hair-like structure, from the placenta and test it. The blood tests and ultrasound combined is 70-90% accurate at predicting whether the Cub will have Down's or another abnormality.

I am opposed to this testing. I think the results will make me more anxious. They are often not correct. And more can be learned at the 20-week, full-body ultrasound than from this early batch of tests. Jim, however, wants to do the NT scan.

I understand his desire to know. He says it will eliminate another worry. I have decided I will go through with the testing, but ONLY if he accompanies me. I will not go alone.

The advantage of knowing about the probability of a genetic disorder is being prepared. If we know in advanced our child could need special care, we can become educated on the disorder. Otherwise, there is no reason for me to know.

Meanwhile, I am investing in a home Doppler. That way, I can hear the Cub's heartbeat any time I want. It may sound extreme, but after what happened with my brother's baby, it would make me feel so much better. My sister-in-law noticed Dylan was moving a little less, but if she had had a Doppler, she would have been able to collect data on him. The same thing happened with Nicholas, too. If I would have been able to hear his heart beating, I would have been able to keep up with his health.

For all its benefits, technology has made pregnancy far more complicated than it was the first time and the second time I was pregnant. I guess much changes in twenty years.

Off to bed to read a book to the Cub. Tonight, we are reading one of my favorites, *Sammy the Seal*.

October 2010

Reading, Writing, and Reassurance

October 4, 2010 at 7:50 pm

EVERY NIGHT WHEN we go to bed, I read a book to the Cub. My favorite book so far is called Dragon's Fat Cat. It is about a blue dragon who adopts a homeless, fat cat (an overweight feline, not an politician). Later, he discovers that the cat, named Cat, is pregnant. Dragon keeps her and her kittens, giving up his own beastly comforts for his new family. I identify with my new, blue friend.

An excellent read!

When we decide to create family, we give up much in the hopes of gaining even more. We create families in multiple ways, and for awhile, my husband believed that our family would be just the four of us (me, him, and our two kitties). And now our baby is on the way. My friends who are parents keep telling me to enjoy these childless moments, and believe me, I do, but I look forward to fall walks through the Big Woods with our child and trick-or-treating (dressed up as a lion, of course). I know, though, that raising a child is more than just happy times, but difficult, challenging moments in which I must put his or her needs before my own.

Of course, all of us moms (and moms-to-be) know that our sacrifices for our children begin even before we get pregnant. We change our diets, stop smoking, stop drinking alcohol, and give up caffeine. But I have happily changed my lifestyle to play my part in bringing a healthy child into this world.

I had a little bit of cramping and spotting today. I reached out to my online support group, and they reassured me that all is more than likely well. More than half of us have experienced spotting and/or cramping in early pregnancy. I have twice and the Cub is always doing well when we take a peek. Although the sight of that bit of pink on the toliet paper has sent me into sheer panic in weeks past, this time, I worried for about an hour and then let it go. I know I cannot change the outcome of this pregnancy. I know I can't close my eyes and wake up with a healthy baby in my arms.

But it surprises me that this moment, during this pregnancy, is the occasion for me being able to let go.

If you have been reading along for awhile, you know that I have been challenged by letting go or letting it be, as the Beatles crooned all those years ago. And yet when I finally admit that I am powerless over my situation, I have no choice but to hope for the best and see what happens.

I have a long way to go before I see my baby's face, before I hold him or her in my arms, before I kiss him or her goodnight. Until then, I will keep on believing that all will be well, making room in my life and in my heart for this Cub I already love deeply. And like Dragon, I am more than prepared to give up my bed and my dinner for the Cub. It is the least I can do for a little being who has already given me more than I can say.

Being in the World

October 7, 2010 at 10:01 am

TIME SEEMS TO BE creeping along. I will be 10 weeks pregnant tomorrow, and it feels like I have been pregnant for much longer. Pregnancies have their way of seeming unending, so I know that I still have a long, long way to go.

I am working from home today after a really long day at work yesterday. The Cub and I need some time in our favorite chair with a stack of student papers and a cup of cocoa. I try to rest as much as I can, but life drags me on. I think sometimes about women who work in fields or factories or under dangerous conditions while pregnant. Somehow they manage and go on to have healthy babies. I guess humans are just destined to go on, at least for awhile longer.

The other day I was walking through the parking garage after work. It had been a long hard day, and I was feeling stressful and tired. I thought I parked on level four, but I was really on level five. As I grumbled about the far walk to the top, a bird tweeted next to me and flew ahead to land on my car. I wondered to myself if this was some kind of sign, given that there were many cars to choose from. Why my car?

As I got closer, I could see the bird's tail feathers. The tips were highlighted with bright yellow. I had never seen this particular kind of bird. As I inched closer, the bird started singing and staring at me. He or she did not move, even after I was close enough to pet it. I didn't, of course. I simply introduced myself and waited for the bird to fly away. After a few minutes of singing and spreading his or her tail feathers, he or she flew off into the sky.

Getting so close to a wild creature is always miraculous to me. I feel as though I am being singled out. That for one moment nature is choosing me because I respect and treasure the inhabitants of our world. Of course, I know that I am giving this bird (and me) to much credit, but one thing is certain: I ended my work day frustrated and depleted and the presence of this lovely bird, a cedar waxwing, made me feel peaceful and happy.

Another lesson in the importance of BEING in the world. The world is full of mysteries and magic. It is our job to seek them out, especially in our times of need.

Wake of Mourning

October 8, 2010 at 9:34 am

...IS THE TITLE OF a poem I wrote about my daughter's death. It detailed the harrowing moments immediately following her murder, but in a partially fictional way. It had big metaphors and seemed removed from the real sadness and grief that persisted for years after I buried her. Now, nearly twenty years later, it is obvious that the "I" in the poem is clearly not me, but someone else: a writer/mother who was afraid to deal with the anguish and grit of loss. I feel sad for her as I do for the dozen or so women in my online support group who lost their pregnancies yesterday.

I have been a member of the site, FertilityFriend.com, since 2003. I enter my ttc data there, and their software processes it and tells me what I need to know about my cycles. By far, though, the best part about FF is the communities—online groups that support each other through trying to get pregnant and the aftermath. My group, May Due Date Buddies, has been in place since right before I found out I was pregnant.

Being a member there is mostly a wonderful help. My paranoias about all things pregnancy can be dismissed by posing a question to all of the other women who are at my stage of pregnancy. We have all had multiple experiences with ttc, pregnancy, and many of us, child loss. I learn a lot from those women and appreciate their willingness to help me and others as we struggle through the fears of bringing a baby home.

Yesterday, however, was brutal.

One after another after another: "I'm out." "It's over." We all responded with sad posts, but the gravity of so many losses of so many women who are at similar stages in pregnancy just confirmed how fragile and fleeting life is.

It took me most of the afternoon and part of the evening to shake off the anxiety that I might be next. It helped that one of my friends on the list talked to me directly. But the shadow of those losses hangs over my growing belly like a dark cloud. It is not nearly as ominous as it was last night, but I believe all of our cores were shaken by the rash of miscarriages in a single eight hour period.

I am turning my focus away from the blackness of loss and to the growing possibilities of life. I am ten weeks pregnant today and despite minor spotting, all has been quite well with me and the Cub. I just have to remember that as much as I mourn on behalf of my group members, they, like the girl in my poem, are not me. My Cub and I are fine. We are going to be fine. We will prevail.

I Look Pregnant!

October 9, 2010 at 10:48 am

YESTERDAY, I WAS having some severe pain in my lower pelvic region. I assumed that it could be round ligament pain (the round ligaments hold the uterus in place), but it seemed way too early! I mean, 10 weeks?!?! So, I called my doctor, and she called me back and asked me if I recently had a uterine growth spirt, and I said, "Yes, all day people have been telling me that I look pregnant." She confirmed that I was indeed experiencing round ligament pain and that it was normal. She also said that part of the pain might be from adhesions that resulted from the placental abruption and c-section with my son. I was so relieved. She told me to take Tylenol and enjoy my weekend.

Indeed, my profile has changed. I now have a round baby bump that is obvious to even not-so-nibby folks. Who knew you could "show" at 10 weeks?

P.S. I love it!

Of Dune Buggies and Uterus-Seat Drivers

October 10, 2010 at 10:55 am

I HAD A STRANGE DREAM last night. I offer it here without analysis. I have too many papers to grade to ponder anything else at the moment.

I am about six months pregnant, and I decided to take a dune buggy to work. I live an hour from home, all interstate. (!!) Anyway, 15 minutes into our return trip home, it begins to rain, hard, so I get out of the buggy and put up a wind/rain shield to protect us from the downpour. A fellow driver (a man in a pickup truck) stops to assist me and to give me some extra gas.

I get back in the dune buggy and the Cub starts complaining: You know, Mom, I told you we shouldn't have taken the dune buggy today. It looked like rain this morning. You should have watched the Weather Channel. And on and on and on.

I am laughing and driving the dune buggy at top speed, which is about 30 mph. (The speed limit on the WV side of I-70 is 70 mph.) As we trundle along with cars passing us and blowing our little buggy all over the highway, the Cub continues his/her rant: I mean, I don't mind so much because I am dry in here, but dang, you must be getting soaked out there. Maybe we should pull over. Do you think we should call AAA? I mean, they might come pick us up.

On our way down 3-mile hill, the wind/rain shield blows off and the Cub and I are without any kind of coverage. All of a sudden, the Cub giggles.

Then, I woke up.....

Scared

October 14, 2010 at 9:35 am

I STARTED HAVING cramping last night. A little bit of spotting turned into heavier spotting. And this morning I passed a small clot.

Praying that it is not over. Praying that I have made it this far and all is still well with the Cub.

HELP!

On Being a Mom

October 14, 2010 at 12:56 pm

I GO IN FOR AN ULTRASOUND tomorrow morning at 8:45. They are usually good at getting me in the same day, but one of their technicians is out sick. I could go to the ER, but I want to see my own doctors. If the news is bad, I want to get it from someone I know.

I had spotted a bit of bright red blood on Saturday, but my doctor said it was nothing to worry about. Then, last night the crampy contractions began. And just as I arrived at work this morning, I felt sick. I went to the bathroom and found quite a bit of pink/red/brown blood on the tp and then passed a black clot the size of an eraser head. Obviously, I freaked out.

I called my doctors immediately and when they called me back, they were not reassuring. They said it didn't sound good.

I know that this could be something called a subchorionic hematoma (a blood clot in the womb), but the contractions make me think it is a miscarriage.

I cried all the hour drive home, unable to live with the possibility that the Cub is not going to make it. Unable to cope with the reality that he/she very well might not.

Tonight, I will read Guess How Much I Love You to the Cub at bedtime. Of course, he/she never has to guess! I love this baby with endless devotion. I just hope that when we do the scan tomorrow, I get to see his/her heart beating again. But a part of me thinks that we might be too late.

Fear of the Unknown

October 14, 2010

MY HUSBAND IS HOME. He hates doctors, especially the ER. He wants me to go get it checked now.

I am afraid.

I don't think I am ready to find out that the Cub is dead.

I just don't know if I can take the news.

I know that might not be the outcome, but if it is, I just don't think I am ready to hear it.

Oh Yes, the Cub Lives!

October 14, 2010

I AM HAPPY to say, the Cub is fine!! We looked at the Cub, measuring 11 weeks and 3 days (four days ahead of schedule). Heartbeat a stunning 173! Everything looked good. My cervix is closed. The bleeding has turned brown.

So far, so good. I go in for a follow up with my doctor tomorrow. I really hope they can figure out why I keep having spotting.

They saw no chorionic hematoma.

The best part was seeing the Cub boogying down to some fetus-frequency music. The second best part was my husband was there to see it!

Two-Week Wait

$%#^&!!

October 16, 2010

Less than 24 hours ago, I got a clean bill of health from my specialist. I had a second ultrasound and a second pelvic exam. The bleeding had stopped, my cervix was closed, and the Cub was doing awesome! This morning: red spotting.

What in the &^%$ is going on? I know that this is not normal. And yet the Cub continues to thrive.

I wish, wish, wish that I could not be alarmed by seeing blood, but I can't. At this point, I know that the chances of having a miscarriage are less than 10%. I have seen the Cub on ultrasound six times. Every single time, the Cub has been doing very well, never dating behind or even on time, but ahead.

So, now my fear is that the bleeding, if it is coming from my uterus, will cause the Cub harm. If it is coming from the placenta it could cause growth retardation. I know I cannot do anything to change the outcome. I know it! And yet I cannot get it off my mind when it is brought to my attention every time I go to the bathroom. (And when you're pregnant, that is about 12x a day.)

I meditate every night and every morning. I do light yoga in the evenings. I listen to positive, relaxing music. And often I am calm and happy. But then I see the spotting, my face falls, and my chest tightens.

I feel so frustrated and worried. I want the Cub to be healthy. I want to stop worrying.

Looking Towards the Future

October 17, 2010

Now everything seems fine with the Cub, I can't help but think ahead a little to the future. I know from experience parenting is not always a happy time (to say the least), but I do know there are many wonderful moments to be had. I am sharing some of those future moments with all of you, since so much lately has been sad.

I look forward to...

1. Looking into the Cub's eyes for the first time. When I finally get to see that sweet face, I know it will take my breath away.
2. Nursing the Cub for the first time. Bonding with the Cub in that special way is important to me.
3. Spending the summer with the Cub. Few working mothers get the opportunity to spend four months with their newborn babies.
4. Taking the Cub trick-or-treating next year. The Cub will be about six months old and dressed as a lion cub (what else!?).
5. Feeding the Cub his first serving of mashed sweet potatoes at Thanksgiving.

I especially look forward to reading bedtime stories to the Cub. I can't wait!

Lately, I have been reading Halloween and Thanksgiving books to the Cub, but last night, we read *Children Make Terrible Pets* by Peter Brown. It is hilarious. Basically, a girl bear cub adopts a little boy that she finds wandering in the woods. It turns out the boy (she names him Squeak) doesn't make a very obedient pet. The main message is that wild animals make poor pets and are probably missed by their families of origin. A good read, even Jim said so.

Tonight, we are digging into one of my favorite books, Sammy the Seal. I guess we shall see if it stands the test of time.

It feels so good to be out from under the cloud of fear for a while. The first trimester screening for birth defects is coming up in nine days. (They re-scheduled it.) I plan on not worrying about that until I get the results, which will be the same day.

Did I mention just how much I love the Cub?

The NT Scan Looms

October 24, 2010

OUR FIRST ROUND of genetic screening is coming on Tuesday. We are both worried, but he is far less worried than me, which is good. One of us needs to at least appear sane.

I have read enough about this particular test to know it might make us more anxious than anything else. Basically, they take a bit of blood from me and create a ratio of hCG (the pregnancy hormone) and PAP-A (another pregnancy-related substance), and then look at a very detailed scan of the Cub. In particular, they look at the nuchal fold thickness (on the back of the baby's head) and the nasal bone (absent or present). From the data they gather, they give me the odds of having a child with certain genetic disorders, including Down's syndrome and spina bifida.

At my age, we have about 1/220 chance of having a child with Down's. As for the other problems, we won't know until after the scan.

Jim is far more optimistic than I am. He thinks "just fine" odds are 1/12, whereas doctors push for chorionic villus sampling (CVS) or amniocentesis if your rate is better than 1/150 or 1/200. (That is to say, 1/100 or something.) Without any further info, we know from research that our chance of having a child free of genetic problems is about 99.5%. Jim is right. Those are pretty good odds.

IN ANY CASE, what will happen on Tuesday is we will go in for the blood test, then the ultrasound. They will give us the results that day. If the results are unfavorable, they will suggest CVS. It will be done that day. I would rather not do CVS because, like amnio, it has a risk of miscarriage.

So much to think about. I just can't wait to see the Cub again on the big screen. The last time, he looked like a cute teddy bear.

Maybe this time, he'll be reading *The Grapes of Wrath* and eating a plum. (Of course, I don't remember putting a fetus-sized novel in there, but you never know....) Have I mentioned how deliriously in love with this Cub I am?

Tonight, we are reading a standard, *If You Give a Cat a Cupcake*.

NT Scan Results

October 26, 2010

I HAD MY NT scan today, too. All looks good.

Measuring a little ahead (13w1d), but not enough to change my due date. Nuchal fold measures: 1.88, which is good. There was a nasal bone.

My odds (I am 37) for Down's: 1/4,100

My odds for Trisomy 18: 1/91,155.

Baby was not as rambunctious as before, but s/he was moving around in there plenty. HB: 158.

Also, I was worried, especially given the spotting, that I had a low lying placenta. They looked and it is just fine. Nowhere near my cervix. Given that was largely the cause my son's death, this was a big relief.

The next testing is between 16 and 18 weeks for spina bifada. Then, a full body scan at 20 weeks.

It was wonderful to see the Cub again.

Lucky Signs

October 30, 2010

I ROUTINELY BUY children's books at the thrift store, though I do buy my share of new books, too. I usually get them for a dime or a quarter, depending on the store. A couple of weeks ago, I bought a dozen new books, mostly storybooks, but a few chapter books that seemed good, including *Who Stole Halloween?* It turns out the mysterious disappearance of a cat named Halloween wasn't the only surprise between the pages.

The other night after I finished carving my pumpkin, I was flipping through the book when I found a mint, crisp $2 bill between pages seven and eight! I took this as a bit of good luck. After all, it wasn't a bill due for $2. I realized, of course, some child probably received the money as a gift and tucked it away in the book for safe keeping. Returning it to its owner would be impossible, so I decided to put it back inside for the Cub to discover some fall afternoon. It will be years from now until s/he is capable of reading this book, so I will have to wait until then to see the Cub's reaction.

Meanwhile, all is well in Cub land. We are hanging in there and enjoying finally being able to relax now that the spotting has stopped and our first round of tests have come back good.

Tomorrow is my birthday. Look for a birthday entry. Don't worry, though, even though I am a Halloween child, it won't be scary. Well, not too scary.

Birthday O'Ween

October 31, 2010

I AM NEARING the end of my 37th birthday. I had a great weekend. I spent time with my husband and with my friends as usual, but this birthday was different than any I have had in nearly a decade. For the first time since 2000, I did not cry on my birthday.

I always enjoyed most of every birthday I have had. What's not to like? Cake AND Halloween candy! But after my son died, each birthday seemed unbearable. Not only did I miss him and my daughter, but the weight of my advancing age on my fertility became harder to deny with each passing year. Then, when I lost my pregnancy in 2004, then the cats to the house fire just months later, and then another pregnancy in 2006, it started to become less and less likely I would ever bring home another child.

In addition, being born on Halloween has its complications for a childless mother. In the US, Halloween is a child's holiday. Everywhere I looked I would see little people dressed in costumes with their parents in tow. And as each year went by, I couldn't stop thinking of my own children and how they would never enjoy this holiday. Beyond that, as much as I tried to participate in Halloween festivities, I was continuously reminded of how much I was missing and of what I may never be able to partake in.

Throughout the years, I borrowed other peoples' children for trick-or-treating. Niece and nephews and the children of friends, and we always had a good time, but the absence of my own little person to dress up and share the day with made me sad. Not only was another year of my life passing, but another Halloween without a child was gone as well.

This year, however, was my best birthday in a long time. Not only did I have a good time with my husband at my favorite restaurant, but I also bought the first piece of furniture for the Cub and I went trick-or-treating with friends and their daughters.

I bought a beautiful gliding love seat for the master bedroom. Since most of the first year of the child's life will be spent in our bedroom, I wanted to get a glider rocker, but the furniture saleswoman showed me a glider sofa, and I was immediately sold. It can easily go from a place to rock and breastfeed to a place to a read a book to the Cub as s/he grows.

I know I should hold off on buying furniture for the Cub, but the nesting impulse is so strong. It really kicked in after the NT scan, especially since I found out the placenta is in the right place. I plan on holding off until after the 20 week full body scan before I buy anything else, but I just couldn't resist this cute little rocker.

Instead of being filled with longing and absence this birthday, I was filled with hope for the future. My spotting has finally stopped, the baby is healthy and strong, and this time next year, I will be taking my sweet Cub out trick-or-treating. Dressed as a lion cub, of course.

Perhaps I am allowing myself to ignore the things that could still go wrong, but I can't help but believe for the first time in this pregnancy that all is well and will be well. The Cub is coming home. No more childless birthdays. No more Halloweens without a Cub.

I believe the power of positive thinking helped us to conceive, and I believe the power of positive thinking (yours and mine) will bring this Cub home safe and sound.

As the last few hours of my birthday come to pass, I am smiling and taking my first peek at ways to put together the nursery. There will be hard days ahead after the Cub comes. I am sure of that. But I also know I will never spend another birthday crying over my rapidly shrinking fertile window.

Happy Halloween everyone! The Cub was going to dress up as a vampire, but he was concerned about the fangs poking me in the uterus (the Cub's considerate). Instead, s/he went as him/herself: a lime-sized gummy bear.

"I can't stop lovin' that [Cub] of mine."

November 2010

The Angle of the Dangle

November 2, 2010 at 9:05 am

MY ONLINE SUPPORT group for nervous pregnant women is having a good time with the images of our NT scans. According to several theories, you can make a pretty good guess about your baby's sex by measuring the angle of the dangle.

According to some research, if the baby's genital "nub" is pointing more than 30 degrees away from the spine, then it is a boy. If the nub is less than a 30 degree angle from the spine, then the baby is a girl. So, I eagerly posted pics from my last scan. The picture is pretty blurry, but according to 99% of my support group, it's a boy!! Pretty darned exciting. I think the baby is a boy and have thought so from about six weeks on, but only time will tell.

What I didn't realize until the other day is that "the angle of the dangle" is part of a pretty filthy axiom: The angle of the dangle is equal to the heat of the meat. Physicists! Obviously, that is a completely different way of looking at the phrase.

In any case, I had a terrible nightmare about the Cub last night that I am still trying to shake, so posting his? pics makes me smile. We should get a better sex prediction at the 20 week full body scan. Still think this Cub is a boy.

Cubdate

November 5, 2010 at 2:33 pm

I HAD MY REGULAR OB appointment yesterday, and all is well in Cubland. Nice, strong heartbeat (158.5 bpm), and moving around like a break dancer. I am 14 weeks pregnant today. The Cub will come into this world in 22 weeks!

I talked to my doctor about everything that has been on my mind lately, including when the Cub would make an appearance. He said between 36 and 37 weeks, which is not all that far from now. So exciting. The Cub's due May 6, but will show up around the second or third week of April. An exact date will be set in the coming months. Needless to say, I am very excited.

I plan on getting started on the nursery over Christmas break and hope to be finished by the end of spring break. I will teach (if all goes well) until a day or two before the expected C-section, which will take me up almost to the end of spring term.

The Cub and I will have nearly five months off together. We can bond and hang out and all those sleepless nights won't be nearly as bad if I don't have to go in to work.

I have three more tests on deck: 1. early glucose tolerance test (Tuesday), 2. a blood test for spina bifida (@16-17 weeks), and 3. the full body scan (@ 20 weeks). We're moving right along.

I hope the Cub enjoys the symphony because that is where we are headed this evening.

Nesting Has Come Home to Roost

November 7, 2010 at 2:52 pm

AND IT IS DIFFICULT for me to ignore. I know I don't have time right now to paint the Cub's room and do all the shopping and cleaning that needs done, but it is so hard not to get started. I have been sick with a migraine and a stomach yuck for two days, but the lure of making a cute space for the Cub is pressing on me. So, I have started making a list of before-birth must-haves.

I know I won't need the crib until the Cub is six months old or so, but I will need the following items before I see that Cubby face:

- bedside crib for easy breastfeeding and staring at the Cub all night
- diapers (cloth and disposable)
- a Pack-n-Play with a bassinet and changing pad
- a dozen or more onesizies
- car seat/stroller combo
- new camcorder
- baby bathtub
- baby towels and washclothes
- swaddling wraps
- baby wipes
- baby lotion :)
- baby hairbrush and grooming supplies
- bottles and sterilizer
- Baby Bjorn baby carrier (front loaded!)
- diaper bag (I like the diaper backpacks)
- two Boppy pillows (one for upstairs and one for down)
- storage units and new bookshelves for nursery
- clothes hamper for nursery
- baby thermometer and suction tool
- bouncy seat and/or swing

I am sure this list will grow as I grow, but it is a place to start!

We plan on painting the room (with NO VOC paint) over Christmas break. We are down to two colors (apple green and green meadow). We have the jungle theme picked out. (Lions, tigers, and...elephants! oh my!).

Of course, I will be quite a bit happier when my headache goes away and my nose stops bleeding. The joys of pregnancy!! It's all worth it for Cubenstein!

A Letter to Cub

November 10, 2010 at 6:18 pm

Dear Cub,

Well, we have made it to 15 weeks! What a relief! Just 22 or so more weeks to go before you come breaking out and into the world.

I don't have much time to write tonight, but something has been on my mind all day, and I wanted to get it down in print before I forgot.

I know I will not be a perfect mother (that would be kind of creepy), but one thing I want you to know above all else is that I love you unconditionally. You will not be perfect either. You will make mistakes. I will have to punish you. You might even hate me sometimes. But I will go on loving you no matter what.

I might not agree with all of the decisions you make in life, including how you wear your hair or your major in college, but I will love you always. Everyone has deep, dark days, Cub, but you can always count on me to be here for you. You will never be alone as long as I am here on Earth. You might not always want to come to me with your troubles, but I promise that I will do my best to try and understand what hurts your heart when you do.

You, wonderful you, were a very long time in the making, but you are worth the wait. Since the moment I found out your little self was growing inside me, I have told you every night, every morning, and throughout that day "I Love You."

See you soon,

Mama

Maternity Clothes Shopping for Dummies

November 12, 2010

EVEN THOUGH I have been pregnant five times, I have never been able to afford maternity clothes. Now I have a bit of extra dough and only two pairs of pants that fit over my ever-bulging belly, I journeyed out to find some maternity wear the other day with my girlfriends in tow. Fail.

I went to eight stores, two of which said on their websites they stocked maternity clothes. I even went to Old Navy (I never shop there) and came up empty. I found some really ugly stuff at Sears (surprise!) and some skinny maternity jeans (srsly!) at Penney's, but all of it made my self-esteem dip a bit lower than it has been lately. I found some stuff at the Gap that wasn't tacky, but it also was a little small.

So, I went up a couple of sizes in regular clothes, and they looked really awful. Baggy everywhere but the baby area. Frustrated, I bought the Cub a stack of books (including an illustrated version of Robert Frost's "Stopping By Woods on a Snowy Evening"), got myself a smoothie, and put my girlfriend's back in the car. Hrumph!

I can't ever buy clothes online. I am a pear and am hard to virtually dress (and hopefully, undress). After getting advice from my online support group for paranoid moms-to-be, I am heading to Motherhood Maternity over Thanksgiving break.

I did buy a pair of jeans that are two sizes bigger than my pre-pregnancy size, but the dumpy butt and baggy legs are well compensated for because they have sparkles on the pocket...

I wonder what I will look like at eight months? I already have a belly. I guess I am going to have to come out at work when we go back in January. Surprisingly, no one has asked me directly. I wouldn't lie about it, of course, but I still want to keep the Cub unofficial until next term. I will have only three months or so of work and then the Cub will arrive. I am guessing it is going to go quickly by the time mid-January rolls around.

Meanwhile, my nephew Dylan, who you may remember was born premature not long ago, will get out of the hospital next Wednesday. He weighs five pounds and is doing quite well! And!!! I got to talk to my nephew on the phone tonight. It is rare. Both are wonderful blessings.

Tonight, the Cub and I are reading *Millions of Cats*. What? The Cub, yeah, the Cub, picked it out.

Worries, Worries, Worries All Day Long

November 18, 2010

"WILL MY PROBLEMS work out right or wrong?" What? I am an Everly Brothers fan. Can you dig it?

Today has been quite a day. I didn't get much sleep last night because of a loud windstorm, and I spent part of the day in a fog. But I feel better than I have in ages, so I can't complain about that.

Then, my sister-in-law called with a big surprise. My nephew Dylan was coming home after being in NICU for two months! I got to hold him for the first time. It was wonderful.

And hanging over my head ... week 16.

I begin week 16 this coming Friday. It is a good thing, progressing well, but it is also a cause for fear. I had my first major bleed with Nicholas during week 16. Even though the reason for that bleed (complete placenta previa) is not an issue with this pregnancy, I just can't help but feel anxious as the week approaches.

That night over nearly ten years ago to the day, blood gushed out of me and onto the chair and floor. I rushed to the ER, and they sent me home, saying that it was the placenta righting itself. Just eight weeks later, the placenta completely abrupted and Nicholas was born at 24 weeks. He only lived a week.

But this upcoming week's worry is not just about the past, but also about the present. On Tuesday of next week, I go in for another round of blood tests. This time to test for neural tube defects, like spina bifida. I am more worried about the results of this round of tests than any of the others because metformin, the drug used to treat Polycystic Ovarian Syndrome, is known to cause B vitamin deficiencies, which can lead to neural tube defects. I did take mega B vitamins, including extra folic acid for more than a year before I got pregnant, so I am hoping I stopped this from happening, but I am still worried about the Cub developing this set of serious problems.

Nonetheless, my doctor reminded me that after a positive pregnancy test, it is too late to do anything about neural tube defects. I really hope the Cub is okay.

Most of the time I am confident all is well, especially since I have had no spotting in more than three weeks. In fact, I have a painter/wall paper hanger guy coming over to help us work out the details of the Cub's room. I am already starting on a registry. And my BFF is planning my shower for mid-March. I mean, I am so excited about this Cub's arrival and usually quite sure that all is well in Cubland, but the gnawing voice in the back of my head speaks from a place of knowledge, an awareness that anything can still happen.

My sister-in-law said when I told her we won't know the gender until around Christmas that "your pregnancy is taking forever!" To me, it seems to be picking up speed. Before I know it, this Cub will be here in my arms, but I am just as happy to have him/her in my belly for the time being. I never have to worry about where he/she is. We are never apart. And that's the way I like it!

Getting Into the Spirit

November 20, 2010

I AM JUST OVER 16 WEEKS today. It is a big relief to have made it this far and all seems well. Of course, because I can't feel the baby move consistently yet, I constantly bug Jim with "Do I still look pregnant?" I suppose the paranoia will never go away entirely, but I am doing what I can to enjoy the second trimester.

Now the sinus infection is gone, I feel better than ever. I plan to take this time (and the break from teaching classes for a week) to get the house ready for Christmas, catch up on grading, and finish revising/writing some projects. Meanwhile, I am working on making a mix CD (formerly known as a mix tape) for Jim for his birthday.

This morning he kept playing the song "Arms Wide Open" by Creed over and over again on his guitar. At some point, he explained it is his way of thinking about and getting in touch with the baby. So, I am going to assemble some songs about fatherhood and give it to him to listen to in his truck on long trips.

I have been given many great suggestions so far, but I am going to wait until after the gender scan (around Dec. 21st) to make the final list.

I had my glucose tolerance test last week, but the results aren't in yet. My next test is blood work for neural tube defects (in three days). I have an OB appointment in two weeks. It is killing me to wait that long. Just dying to checking on the Cub.

Meanwhile, we are still trying to finalize our nursery plans. We have too many good ideas! We know it will be lion themed and will be borrowed from Edward Hicks' *The Peaceable Kingdom*, but beyond that, we are not sure of anything, include wall and wallpaper color.

I was hoping to get that part of it done over Christmas break, but it might not happen...

It is good to finally feel that I can breathe a little bit in this pregnancy. My energy is back, and despite the moments of "Cub, you still there?" I am enjoying getting ready for this baby's arrival. Just 21 weeks left.

Test Results, and Dancing Cub

November 22, 2010

MY DOCTOR'S OFFICE called with my glucose tolerance test (GTT) results: 95! That's good. 135 or over is not good. She said, "Go ahead and have some extra mashed potatoes this year!" I laughed. How did she know that mashed potatoes are my all-time favorite preggo food? (Okay, so they are my all-time anytime food, but I digress...)

I just got back from getting more blood work done: Second Trimester Screening. They test for neural tube defects (like spina bifida), and they also test again for Down's. I am hoping that all will come back good. My nurse's office said I should hear something by Friday/Monday at the latest. I am nervous, but hopefully, the Cubster is super groovy in there.

While signing in at the hospital, the registration clerk asked me if I was carrying any weapons. I laughed and said, "No, but my fetus is." Clearly, she was not amused. However, I could hear the guy waiting in line behind me braying like a donkey. Too funny.

One thing is certain: this baby likes to groove. For three days, the Cub has been rolling around in me like s/he is in the roller derby. It is wonderful to finally feel consistent movements throughout the day. (As I am typing this, my uterine wall is being pummeled by teensie, tiny Cub feet.) If you have never felt the pleasure of baby movement, it feels at first like butterfly wings beating softly inside you. Soon, it becomes more like tumbling, like your dryer has an unbalanced load. (That's the stage I am in right now.) Later, it feels more like a punch or a kick from a tiny person, and it is!! I giggle every time the Cub gets moving in there. I cannot help myself. I love that Cub!

Writing It Out

November 23, 2010

I AM WRITING this entry tonight in the hopes it will help me calm down. I have had cramping and pelvic heaviness for about nine hours. I kept thinking it was from walking earlier today or from not drinking enough water, but no matter what I do or don't do, it is there.

I have talked to my support group gals about it, and they are convinced it's a normal part of the growing process. However, it is freaking me out. It is not painful at all, just stronger than the usual aches and pains I have had throughout this pg.

Of course, I am obsessively checking to see if I am spotting again and all is good there, but now I wish I would have called my doctor earlier. I could still call, but what would I even learn if I called at 11:30 at night?

If the discomfort is still there in the morning, I will call.

It's going to be hard to sleep, especially since I am home alone again tonight.

I met Jim for dinner this evening, and we were talking about the baby. He was so excited, but I was holding back because I could feel the cramping and heaviness. I haven't felt the baby move today. I know that is not unusual at all for this stage of pregnancy.

I sure hope it is just a bad case of gas.

Heading to the Doctor

November 24, 2010

I CALLED MY DOCTOR to ask about the cramping and pelvic heaviness, and she is pretty sure that it is bowel related or from the movement of my uterus from my pelvic region to my abdomen. In any case, she wants me to come in for my own piece of mind. I guess all the doctors in that practice know that I am a nervous, preggo lady.

In any case, I am about to hear the Cub's heartbeat. I would shut my big toe in a car door to see his/her little face again, but I am betting I will only get to hear some little bitty heart thump, thump, thumping away, which is just fine with me!

Full report on my return.

Cub News

November 24, 2010

MY FAVORITE DOCTOR wasn't in today, so I had to see another doctor in the practice. The Cub has a great heartbeat (147 bpm) and my cervix is closed, which means the Cub isn't coming out any time soon. My blood pressure is great at 112/73.

She thinks that it was intestine related. She said I shouldn't worry about it. She did say, though, she was glad I came in to see her because it is always good to get discomfort checked out.

The weirdest thing that happened: she told me to gain some weight! Now, I am a pretty plump gal, and my actual doctor in the practice told me to gain a total of 15 pounds throughout the whole pregnancy. I have gained about six so far. That has been intentional. I still consume the recommended daily allotment of calories for a pregnant woman, but I make sure I don't overindulge. I don't want to get gestational diabetes or pregnancy-induced hypertension. I want to have a healthy pregnancy.

I have never had anyone in my entire life recommend that I gain weight. Odd. I will ask my doctor about this when I see him on Thursday of next week. I am guessing he will still stand by his recommendation.

I guess I must stop worrying. The Cub's good. My cervix is good. I just wish I knew for sure that things would stay this way.

A Little Bit Nervous

November 28, 2010

MY DOCTOR'S OFFICE said the test results from the 2nd trimester screening should be back by tomorrow, and I am really nervous about the results. It could change our risk of Down's syndrome and reveal neural tube defects. I am not going to obsess over it, and I am wondering if I should call and ask or just wait for them to call me? I am not good at waiting, but not knowing bad news gives me more time to just be a normal pregnant chic.

I have a Cub doc appointment this Thursday, and I have a ton of questions to asking, including: why is pregnancy filled with aches and pains. I feel like my uterus is colicky. Blah!

In other news, we should find out if the Cub is doing just as expected when we go in for the scan during Christmas week. I am going to try to get the appointment for hubby's birthday. What a wonderful gift! We will also find out the gender that day, which I plan to announce on a cake at Christmas dinner. And, of course, right here.

17 weeks and two days today! Less than 20 weeks left until I see my Cub's stunning face. I wonder if I will ever get back to the point of relaxing and enjoying this pregnancy. I sure hope so because it was a lot more fun when I wasn't worried so often.

I Imagine...

November 29, 2010

I imagine the moment
when the cacophony of the delivery room
blurs into the background,
and they place my child's squirming body on my bare chest.
I imagine him or her suckling at my breast
and gripping my finger in his or her tiny hand.
I imagine those first few moments when I meet this child,
already so loved. Already so anticipated.
These imaginary landscapes propel me onward
when the fear of child loss once again bears down on me.
I am so sure that this baby will come home in my arms
that I have given my heart no other alternative
than to accept a lifetime of unconditional love
that began long before this child was in my womb.
I imagine you, Cub,
your tiny face and bright eyes
squinting at the glaring hospital lights,
trying so hard to catch a glimpse of your Mama,
whose voice you will already know.
I imagine you, Cub,
feeling the warmth of my gentle hands
on your newborn back as I cradle you outside my body
for the first time.
I imagine you, Cub,
as the wonderful being you are,
filling the void that was long ago left in my life
and creating a world that is of your own making.

Second Trimester Screening Results

November 30, 2010

AFTER A WEEK of chewing on my fingernails, I finally heard from my doctor's office. My second trimester screening results came back normal for neural tube defects. So, as far as these blood results go, the Cub is healthy and just dandy in there.

I am incredibly relieved. I was worried about these results more than any other because of being on Glucophage (metformin) for so long. It is known to deplete the body of B vitamins. Low levels of folic acid have been proven to cause neural tube defects, like spina bifida.

I have a regular OB appointment on Thursday. I get to hear Cub's heartbeat then, but I sure wish I could take a nice peak. Hearing the heartbeat is wonderful, but seeing that squirming Cub groovin' out in there is so much better.

I will also be scheduling an appointment for my 20 week anatomy scan, where we will get to see how the Cub is doing and get to know if it is a boy Cub or a girl Cub. What a wonderful Christmas gift! And I plan on scheduling it for Jim's 50th birthday.

Until then, I just have to rely on feeling the Cub rolling around in there and hearing his/her heartbeat every three or four weeks.

December 2010

The Cub is . . . Cubzilla!

December 2, 2010 at 1:41 pm

I WENT TO MY regular ob appointment this afternoon to check in on the Cub. The doctor tried to find the Cub's heartbeat with a handheld Doppler, but could not. However, the Cub was kicking that Doppler like crazy! Even the doctor was amazed at how strong the Cub is at this point. He kept saying, "Wow! Did you feel that?!?!" Of course I did!! The Cub is kicking the inside of ME! Hence, the Cub is Cubzilla today. Taking down Dopplers with a single kick!

Nonetheless, the doc had to get out the ultrasound machine, which didn't disappoint me one bit. I got to see the Cub!! The problem was that the Cub is four and a half inches (the doc measured it) from my skin, which made hearing the heartbeat impossible with a Doppler. The Cub was kicking up a storm in there. I got to see the top of the Cub's head, an arm, and a tiny Cub hand. It was wonderful. Oh, and the heartbeat: 145 bpm. Perfect! (BTW, in case you are wondering, the Cub weighs in at about 6 ounces right now. Itty bitty Cubby.)

He told me I was doing very well. My blood pressure is normal at 116/74 and my weight is good, too. He did, though, remind me that I am at high risk of pre-term labor because of what happened with Nicholas. Of course, this freaked me out, but he reminded me that there is nothing anyone can do to stop that from happening, especially if I have an abruption. I have a 1 in 10 chance of having another abruption. Believe me, I do not want that to happen again.

He also told me that he understands why I am anxious about the baby. He says that daddies never really truly know what moms go through while pregnant. The attachment that moms have long before dads ever do makes some of us go a little crazy with worry from time to time. I was glad he said that. I needed to hear it because sometimes I don't think anyone understands why this pregnancy is so scary for me.

But I am turning my focus to the now. Right now, this baby is healthy. I am healthy (all but a sore throat). I cannot dwell on what may be. After all, I have a 90% chance of not having an abruption. I must look on the positive side.

We go in to get a close up of the Cub on Jim's 50th birthday. I cannot wait to get some good feedback from the scan and to find out if the Cub is a boy or a girl. It is hard to see the Cub on ultrasound because I so want to take him/her out of there and hug him/her tight. But until that day comes, I must be content with grey and white images and the sound of a heartbeat calling me to believe that all will be well.

We're Halfway Home!

December 6, 2010 at 6:11 am

AS OF TODAY, we are halfway to the Cub's birthday! The Cub will be born through mandatory c-section between 36 and 37 weeks of pregnancy, which means that at 18w3d we are at the midway point!

By the time the new semester begins in January, we will nearly be in the third trimester. It won't be long before this Cub is in my arms. Time has gone by more quickly since the spotting stopped.

The fear of seeing that blood day in and day out was enough to stop time.

I am at that wonderful stage of pregnancy where the baby is moving, but I am not uncomfortable all the time. I had terrible right-sided pain all night Saturday night, but it was just round ligament pain. The Cub is clearly growing.

As much as I look forward to seeing my Cubby's face, I can wait until s/he is done growing inside me. It sure is tough, though!

Dealing with Loss that is Not Your Own
December 10, 2010 at 5:52 pm

THIS WEEK WAS a troubling week for a variety of reasons. One of our college students was killed, my brother's baby was falsely diagnosed with meningitis, and my husband and I have been struggling with communication issues. In addition, one of the women in our support group lost her baby at 16 weeks gestation. That loss has had a near-crippling effect on all of us.

Medical journals and internet sites declare that after the first trimester is over, then the risk of miscarriage drops significantly. In fact, these materials make it seems that once a pregnant woman hits 13 weeks, she is in the clear. Unfortunately, I know better than some how untrue this really is. Many problems can still arise after that first trimester is over. In fact, in some ways, I fear those last 13 weeks far more than the first 13. After all, the risks to the mother's health is greatly increased in that last trimester.

My support group member does not yet know the baby's cause of death, but she carried her little one for two days after its life was extinguished. The anguish of such loss is hard to even consider. We sent comforting words to her, but there is really nothing anyone can do to assuage that kind of grief. For her to have made it that far, three weeks past that seemingly magic turning point, and then to lose her baby . . . is unthinkable.

It shook our little group to its core. Many of us immediately began to wonder if our babies were still alive. What if they died since the last ultrasound? We all know there is nothing that can be done before 24 weeks gestation (and if then, help is limited), but that didn't stop any of us from making frightened calls to our doctor's offices.

I am grateful for the Cub's daily exercise routine. S/he keeps me sane when those movements begin. But even so, I was worried when the Cub didn't seem to move as much as s/he had the day before. I know that the Cub is more than likely fine, but the specter of this support group loss hangs over me as much as my own.

This morning while driving to work, I felt the Cub's first kick of the day. I smiled and said, "Good morning, Cub!" I can't live everyday in fear that something has or will go wrong. I can only live one tiny Cubby kick at a time and be glad of it. But I sure wish I could take the grief away from the other mother her lost her baby long after she had already fallen in love with it's little self.

Making My Wishes Known

December 13, 2010 at 11:58 am

I BEGAN THIS BLOG in March of this year (nine months ago!) with entries about wishing. I read countless books on the proper way to wish, the power of wishing, and the the odds that my wishes would come true. But expressing wishes for the future is not the only kind of wishing that can be done. This weekend I made my other wishes known to my husband. In short, what to do if something happens to me and the Cub.

Talking about your own demise is always difficult, but I believe that it is important for peace of mind. When my daughter Samantha was murdered, I didn't have money for an expensive funeral, so my family decided that she should be buried on top of my grandfather's grave. It gave me great comfort to know that my little girl would share the same resting place with the man who had loved me so much.

When my son died, his father and I decided to bury him in the Fisanick family plot in Pennsylvania. We were living in a college town at the time. It would never be our permanent home. It was important to us that our son be with family. He shares a gravesite with his great uncle, who was a Catholic priest and with whom Nicholas shares his name.

I explained to Jim that if the Cub and I do not survive at any point during the pregnancy or after the birth that we be buried together. He said, "Why?" And I said, "Because the Cub is my child. S/he is part of me now and forever. I don't want to go without him or her."

I know it won't matter. I won't know whether the Cub is with me or not. But knowing that he will fulfill my wishes gives me peace now.

I hope he never has to make such a terrible call, but I can't imagine leaving this world without my Cub.

In happier news…I get to see my lovely Cub in just 10 days. We are incredibly excited to see how big Cub has grown and to see how s/he is doing. And we will probably get a glimpse of boy or girl parts. What a wonderful Christmas present for me, and a great 50th birthday present for Jim. Now, if I can just get the Cub to smile for the camera.....

Surprise Cub Check

December 14, 2010

SOMETHING HAS FELT OFF for the past week. Not with the Cub, but just in the general Cub area. I called my doctor, and he said to come in. Everything's okay, and I got to hear the Cub's heartbeat.

It turns that I was right. My vaginal pH is off by just a fraction (5, normal is 1.3-4.5), but enough for me to notice. He said he was shocked that I even picked up on that, given that it is so subtle. I explained I know my body well and things just didn't seem to be operating as usual.

Although I am glad it is nothing horrible, I am not pleased I have to take Flagyl as a precaution. He is worried that my unbalanced pH might make me susceptible to infection. The Flagyl will take care of that.

Flagyl is the worst drug I have ever taken. This past May it made me have severe joint pain and unbelievable exhaustion. I need my energy more than ever right now, so I am quite worried about the side effects.

Nonetheless, I am going to take it to protect the Cub. There are several kinds of infection that can cause pre-term labor, and I really want to avoid that.

It was worth the two hour roundtrip to hear the Cub's heartbeat today. In the 140s. Love that Cub!

Tomato Vines and Pre-term Labor

December 16, 2010

I HAD A HORRIBLE DREAM last night. It has lingered all day, so I figured I had better write it down.

Right before going to bed last night, I stupidly read a story about a woman who died not long after her son was born. It was actually an interesting piece of writing. Basically, the family agreed to let a national magazine run an annotated conglomeration of the woman's status updates about her pregnancy, the birth, and the complications that followed. (I would post a link, but I can no longer find the article online.)

Guess who had a panic attack right before climbing under the covers?

It is no wonder, then, I dreamed I had tomato vines growing through my uterus and out of my vagina. They bore only half ripe fruit, which I collected in a wooden bowl.

I woke up this morning with sharp, spiking pain in my lower abdomen, so I assumed I must have been having that dream in the night because of the pain. After all, it would hurt badly to have a tomato vine jutting out of your vagina.

Then, after talking about it with Jim, I realized it was more than likely a dream about pre-term labor, which is a real concern for this pregnancy and any pregnancy I may have. The tomatoes were not fully ripe; therefore, premature.

The morning spiking pains lasted for two hours and then turned into what felt like the after effects of doing 100 sit ups. (You're right, I have never done 100 sit ups, but I have done 30....) I still have a bit of heaviness. It was scary. I was worried all day.

I think it was some tearing of scar tissue. That's how it felt. I described this to a friend, and she said, she had the same pain. Sigh.... Pregnancy just isn't easy. But I have to admit that this one is going way better than I expected it would.

Tomorrow, I will be 20 weeks pregnant. It is a major milestone. We have 17 weeks left, and just seven days left until I see the Cub on the big anatomy scan. I cannot wait to see my Cubby. One more week....

The Light at the End of the Tunnel

December 17, 2010

WE HAVE JUST 17 WEEKS to go before Cub comes into this world. When I think about it, I tear up. The idea we could get that far is still overwhelming to me.

I am 20 weeks pregnant today. In a month, the Cub will be considered viable, but Nicholas was born at 24 weeks, and he wasn't even close to viable. I am worried, still. I don't think there is anything that will change that. But I believe we are going to make it.

Cub's big scan is in six days. I am scared and excited. Hopefully, the Cub is completely healthy. All signs seem to show that is the case. I think I will feel even more confident once we get the news all is well.

It is a bit risky to schedule the scan on Jim's 50th birthday, but I am so optimistic that the Cub is healthy, I thought it would be a wonderful way to celebrate! (There will be cake, too.)

Until then, I will continue reading books to my Cub (s/he can hear now!) and doing my best to stay healthy. In a little over four months, the Cub will be in my arms.

Into the Ashes, or Blood Moon Rising

December 20, 2010

TRAGEDY ANNIVERSARIES usually do not pass unnoticed, and this one is certainly no exception. Six years ago this very night my house in Cincinnati burned down, and my six cats perished. I write about it now (again) because I have no choice. I am unable to work on other projects, wrap Christmas presents, or visit with friends. I have tried to look that long ago grief in the face and move on, but like other parts of my past, there are still so many words to say about that freezing winter's night when my world was destroyed.

My then-husband Nick and I had just returned from an early Christmas visit to family in West Virginia. We went early so that we could spend Christmas day with our six cats. They were family to us, as much like children as our own son, Nicholas, who had died in 2001. We got up that morning, suitcases still unpacked from our out-of-town trip, and debated how to spend the day. We

Into the Ashes, or Blood Moon Rising

played with the cats, watched some movies, and around 7 pm decided to go Christmas shopping for each other, a fun chore we put off so that we could exchange gifts after we got home.

We went shopping, had a nice dinner, and headed back to the house to share the spoils of our spree. (Nick got me J'adore perfume, and I got him a science kit he had been wanting.) As we made our way to our little part of the city, I spotted the plume of thick gray smoke curling into the night sky. I KNEW at that moment, still more than five miles away, that our house was on fire; our kitties were dead.

I tried to put it out of my mind, and we stopped at the drugstore to pick up a prescription. While checking out, the cashier said she heard a house in Norwood, our neighborhood, was on fire. I rushed to the car, and we sped home. We rounded the corner to our street and saw the blaze. I screamed and jumped out of the car while it was still moving. I ran on the icy sidewalk to the house. Ran to the scene. Ran to get my kitties out.

I remember screaming their names over and over again as I hurled myself towards the fire engines' flashing lights: "Wladek! Mila! Yoshi! Blackie! Barkley! Snowball!" Over and over again, I cried out their names. Nick parked and chased after me. As we approached the house, our neighbors shouted, "It's them!"

I clutched one of the firemen's heavy jacket and begged him to tell me the news: 'Did you find my babies inside?" He said two of the cats had been pulled out of the blaze. I smiled and kissed him, praying that he was right. Later, I would learn that indeed Snowball and Blackie had been rescued from the house, but they were already dead by that time. We found their bodies on the porch and on the sidewalk. I realized Snowball more than likely died after he got out of the house. He was overcome by the water hoses and froze to death trying to escape.

At that moment, nothing in the world mattered more than them. I tried to run up the steps to the house, but the firemen held me back. I kept screaming, "My babies!" Yes, I was reliving the night my daughter was murdered and the day my son was taken off life support. And yes, I knew my cats had become surrogate children. And I am pretty sure they knew it, too, and did not mind at all.

As they continued to fight the flames, I called my mother and told her the news. I then collapsed into a snow bank, unable to get up for quite some time, my eyes never leaving the burning wreck that trapped my beloved cats inside.

If you have never been close to an animal, then you cannot understand the pain I am feeling or the love I felt every single day I shared my life with them. They all came into my life in many different ways, and the most recent additions (Mother's Day, 2003), Wladek and Mila, were just three HOURS old when we took them in. I bottle fed them and bathed them like I would a newborn, playing out those roles that I missed with my son while he struggled for life just two years before. Nick and I shared these parenting duties, and we kept a journal, which recorded how much they ate and drank and if they peed or not.

By the time of the fire, I was head over heels in love with them, but Wladek and I had a special bond. He slept under my shirt while I was sitting on the couch watching TV, he followed me all over the house, he loved for me to brush his teeth, and he slept with his face on my face every single night I was home. He liked to perch on the living room banister as I recited Elizabeth Barrett Browning's "How Do I Love Thee?" And yet there were always too many ways to count.

I thought his death would kill me. I felt like dying. It was only after I found myself freezing and stunned sitting inside the Red Cross van I realized I had nothing but the clothes on my back and the presents we had just bought each other. I remember asking the Red Cross worker, "What do people do when they have lost everything?"

He paused for a long time and then looked me in the eyes and said, "I don't know."

I was in my third semester of teaching at Xavier University. Nick and I were new in town. We were only mildly acquainted with my colleagues at the University. We were alone in a big city with nothing. Very little money. No family. No good friends. Just a car that barely ran that was now frozen to the cement under the carport where we left it before our trip north. (We had to take a rental car or risk breaking down on the highway.) Needless to say, we had no place to go. We ended up checking into a motel for the night, but of course, no sleep would be had. I never stopped crying and said little more than Wlad's name until my brother arrived at 4 a.m.

At dawn that morning, we went back to the house to search for the cats. I called to them, wailing over the smoke alarm's blare. We could not go in the house. We could not do anything but search the ground, the bushes, and the trees. Other than Blackie and Snowball's bodies, we found no sign of our other cats. I refused to leave the scene... until I lost my voice and could not call to my beloved.

That night, a blizzard hit. Within 48 hours, the city was covered in more than 16 inches of snow. We were catless, homeless, and snowed in.

Thankfully, another professor at the University, a woman I did not know, offered us her home until we found a place to live. Jen will always be an angel to me. She selflessly gave us a place to stay when we were at our lowest point.

A day later, another angel came to our rescue: Jim.

At this point, I had known Jim for 11 years. We had dated for a while in 1996, but broke up. We went back to being friends, best friends. As soon as he heard the news, he drove on unplowed roads for five hours on his birthday to make sure I was safe. He gave us money to get back on our feet. But most importantly, he let me take care of him for a couple of days. I made him a big Christmas Eve dinner, and it was such a comfort to be able to care for him. If he hadn't showed up, I would have spent that day and many days thereafter in bed crying. But he was there, and I had a purpose. I will never, ever forget him for doing that for me. Love can be given in many different ways.

In the days and weeks ahead, my neighbors across the city proved to be incredibly generous. They had a pancake breakfast, collected donations and gave us household goods and food. We were touched beyond measure.

And yet I remained incredibly grief stricken, thinking of little else than my Wlad and his brothers and sister. Those last hours. The fire chief told me repeatedly they would have died quietly from smoke inhalation before they even knew what was wrong, but that was little comfort to me. Even though they found all of the cats' bodies when they went back inside, I believed for months and months after the fire that somehow Wlad had survived. I search and searched for him. I KNEW he was gone, but I couldn't stop looking for my Wlad. Sometimes I wake up looking for him in my bed, on my cheek, but he lives now only in my heart and mind.

And like when my children died, I believed that I was responsible. I had promised my babies, and I had promised my cats that I would protect them, and yet I could save none of them.

Even after we sued and won a suit of negligence against our landlord (he had never properly maintained the furnace), I still spent night after endless night crying and chanting my apologies to my cats, to my daughter, to my son for letting them all down.

Six years later, the horrific pain of that fiery night has lessened, something I truly believed could not happen. I am still afraid of house fires. I am still afraid when I hear a fire engine's wail. I still panic any time Jim lights our fireplace.

We finally adopted more cats, nearly two years after the fire. I sit here with Toby and Ginger on a night much like that night. It is freezing cold, and I have just finished Christmas shopping. I doubt the fear will ever go away entirely. I will never be able to leave my Christmas lights on all night or be able to leave the house without doing several cat headcounts. But I no longer live trapped in the darkness of the longest night of the year.

In fact, for two weeks leading up to the fire, my grandmother, who had died just months before, kept appearing in my dreams. She kept trying to tell me something. I couldn't understand her. Her birthday is on Dec. 21, just one day after the house fire. I have wondered if she was sent to me. I have also wondered if I knew something bad was about to happen. Just a week before I had taken a picture of me and Wlad. I was so sad looking in that picture, but being with Wlad always made me happy. The day of the fire, I woke up with his face on my face like usual, but I remember thinking, "This is the last morning I will wake up with Wlad. This is the last time I will feel his warm breath on my cheek and see his big yellow eyes smile a bright good morning."

I dismissed these feelings (*premonitions* in grandma speak) mostly because I didn't know what to do with the information.

There will be a total lunar eclipse tonight. The first one to fall on the Winter Solstice in 456 years. It won't happen again until Dec. 21, 2094. At its peak (around 3:17 am EST), the moon will appear blood red. According to astrologist Dorothy Morgan,

> *Being that we have this eclipse at the last degree of Gemini and this rules the throat charka some of us may need to make amends, forgive others, or ourselves for past interactions. We are being asked to release our wounds in this regards so we can move forward and not hold on to the past, release past actions, or that of others. Forgiving and saying this is a key component with this eclipse.*

I could choose once again to ignore this premonition, but I think this time I will listen and act. I must forgive myself for Samantha's death, for Nicholas' death, and for my cats' deaths. I must release the past and look to the future: the Cub.

The Cub's scan is just three short days from now. I am hoping with all my heart everything is well. I hope we will get the best news:

the Cub is progressing, his or her little body is perfectly formed, and we can walk out into the cold December afternoon confident that our Cub will be with us in 16 weeks.

Perhaps the understanding of this rare eclipse explained at Astrology-Classes.com fits our situation best:

> *This lunar eclipse asks us to take a long, hard look at the issues in our life that are holding us back or that are keeping us from fulfilling our destiny and to make decisions about a more positive, life-affirming way of meeting those challenges.*

Moving forward into the light of that blood red moon. I'll be up at 3 a.m. telescope pressed to the window in the Cub's room, telling the Cub all about this once-in-a-lifetime eclipse. I will not promise my love that I can always protect him or her. I know now that I CANNOT make that promise. But I will tell the Cub I am letting go of the self-blame. I am letting go of the dread I feel about him or her being born in 2011. Samantha was born and died in 1991. Nicholas was born and died in 2001. This coming decade WILL be different. This pregnancy and birth WILL be different.

On this night, six years after my fur babies died, I will remember them because I cannot forget them. They helped me through some of the worst moments of my life (Nicholas' death, my grandparents' deaths, two miscarriages, and many more travails). I will send them kisses by the light of the red moon and turn towards the future: Cub. Healthy, whole, wonderful Cub.

Father Knows Best

December 22, 2010

I ASKED FOR IT, and I got it. Jim has been reading pregnancy books. Of course, that means that he is daily bestowing his newfound knowledge onto me. And you can imagine how well that is going.

I am quite thankful he has taken an active interest in the baby's growth. It lessens my burden to know someone else has at least a working understanding of all the changes going on inside me and the Cub.

It is quite endearing when he asks if I take my vitamins twice a day instead of just once or if I interact with the baby throughout the day. Of course I do these things. There is not much info he can add to my already vast knowledge of prenatal care, but it is wonderful to be able to have a conversation with him about placental growth or fetal brain development and have him follow along.

Of course, the other night when he came to bed and asked me why I was sleeping on my right side instead of my left, I did feel a little annoyed. When I explained I knew sleeping on my left side was best for the baby, but my left leg fell asleep, he seemed satisfied.

All in all, it is quite a good thing he has taken an interest in the pregnancy.

Tomorrow is the big scan. I am nervous, but trying to think positively. 17 weeks to go.

T-Minus Three Hours and Counting

December 23, 2010

I SLEPT only a little last night, even after I wore myself out making goodies for today's birthday feast for hubby and his family. You would think after making a giant pan of homemade lasagna, which included simmering the homemade sauce for six hours, and making homemade apple pie and shopping for Christmas dinner I would have slept well, but I did not.

I read for hours and finally fell asleep at 1 a.m. I woke up at 5:30 unable to get back to sleep.

In three hours I will know more about the Cub than ever before. I know will know if s/he is healthy in all ways and if s/he is a boy. I just hope that the baby has progressed on track. One more milestone to achieve.

Thank you all for thinking of us today. I will update as soon as I can.

It's a ...

December 23, 2010

...HEALTHY BABY! Thank goodness the Cub is fine. All body parts are measuring exactly in line according to gestational age. We could not get a good view of the heart because the rib cage was casting a shadow, but every other Cubby part looked fantastic. My doctor will likely send me for a follow up ultrasound soon to check on that heart just in case. (Pics to come in future posts, including an excellent shot of a Cub paw.)

I cannot tell you how much better I feel. The Cub was going crazy in there, even drinking amniotic fluid. (Don't worry, that's what fetuses do!) It was a painful, hour-long exam. They had to continuously jab the ultrasound Doppler into my belly button, which hovered over a necessarily full bladder. But it's all worth it.

And now for the big sex reveal. We are having a boy cub. Yep, just like we all thought. I am absolutely thrilled and so is Papa Lion.

I think I can just enjoy this pregnancy now. Of course, it won't be long before I become physically uncomfortable with the weight of this Cubby, but I will just have to suffer through the next sixteen weeks.

Oh, what a wonderful day! And what a great day for Jim to find out that he is having a healthy son—his 50th birthday.

Little Cub Things

December 29, 2010

ON MY WAY HOME from lunch with one of my girls, I decided to stop at the thrift store nearby. I love thrift store shopping, and I figured that maybe I would "look" at some Cub stuff. I ended up buying him two bags of clothes.

I hate paying retail for kid's clothes. It is such a waste because they grow out of them so quickly. And many of the pieces I bought still had their original price tags on them!

As exciting and fun as it was to pick out little clothes for the Cub to wear in about four months, I couldn't help but be reminded of the last time I bought a bunch of baby clothes. It was a decade ago, and I was buying them for my son, Nicholas. One of the hardest parts of coming home after he died was knowing that box of clothes and toys was sitting in the spare bedroom. After a few weeks, I went through them all one more time, sealed the box, and put them away. I kept thinking about how painful that moment was, but I also realized this pregnancy is far different. This boy is already way ahead of Nicholas in terms of growth, and I do not have placenta problems. I'm healthy. Cub's healthy.

I know I will not be able to avoid such bittersweet moments in the future. I am sure that holding my son will bring back memories of my other children, but it is all a part of who I am. The Cub will be his own guy, but I will always look for traces of Samantha and Nicholas in his little face, in his cry, and in his tiny grip.

January 2011

It's Almost Shower Time!

January 3, 2011 at 11:07 pm

OVER THE HOLIDAYS, I had a chance to talk to my friend of ten million years, Diane, about the baby shower. She is leading the charge and planning the event. We have decided on March 19 at 2 pm.

It will be a good day for a shower. It's about a month before Cub comes. We couldn't have it on March 5 because Nicholas was born that day. We couldn't have it on March 12 because Nicholas died that day. So, March 19 is the perfect day to get everyone together to welcome the Cub.

I am working on a registry now, but I really love hand-me-downs and homemade baby stuff. The nursery will be green with a jungle theme. It will be done by the time of the shower.

I am so excited about the shower. My favorite part will be the signing of the Cub's book. I want everyone who has a played a part in his journey to write him a message that he can read someday. (Given that he's my boy that will probably be when he is three months old. LOL)

Nightmares Can Come in Pairs

January 7, 2011 at 1:07 pm

I WONDERED WHEN I would have one like this. I knew it was coming. Last night I dreamed that my water broke and the Cub was coming now—at 23 weeks. I fell back asleep an hour later and the nightmare continued. I never want to fall asleep again.

I am just one week away from the baby being considered viable. That is, if he was born a week from today, then he would have a chance of survival outside of the womb. Not a very good chance, but better than right at this moment. I am also one week away from when Nicholas was born. My anxiety is climbing, but I had no idea how much I must worry about having him so early until the nightmares.

The dream began with me and Jim asleep in a big bed. It seemed as though we were on vacation. It smelled and felt like we were at a hotel at the beach. The romance and pleasure of a pleasant vacation faded quickly when I woke up to my water breaking. At first I was thrilled, and I woke up Jim, saying, "My water broke. Your son will be here soon!" We both smiled, and then I realized that I was only 23 weeks pregnant. I started crying and repeating, "He cannot survive at this age. He is too small."

We found a doctor, who said that the baby would come, and they would "dispose" of him. I freaked out. Wailing, "Why?! Give him a chance to survive! Help him live!" But the doctors were convinced that he would die. Before he could be delivered, I woke up crying.

Thankfully, Jim was home, and he sensed my distress. He folded me up in his arms and patted my Cub spot saying, "See. He's still in there. He's okay."

He left for work about an hour later, and I fell back to sleep. At some point I re-entered the dream.

This time, the doctors were more optimistic. One doctor said, "He was measuring a week ahead. He might be okay." Nothing they did, though, would console me. I knew my son was coming, and it was far too early.

They told me he was coming so early because he had a heart defect, which is the one part of his little body we did not get a clear picture of at the big anatomy scan. His rib cage was in the way, and he would not turn so they could see it. We go for a follow-up in about three weeks. I will be so glad to get confirmation that he is okay. In my nightmare, he was not.

I woke up just as they were wheeling me into the delivery room.

He is okay. I can feel him moving as I type this. I am okay. All but a minor virus this week, I have been fine. I think more of the anxiety will fade after I get past the week that Nicholas was born and died. But then I have to face 27 weeks, when my nephew was born. He is doing far better than expected, but he has a long, long road to go down.

My doctor plans on taking him in 14 weeks. We can make it. I know we can!

"Gently Rapping, Rapping at My Chamber Door"

January 9, 2011 at 8:11 pm

AND THE DREAMS CONTINUE. This one, though, was not a nightmare. Rather, it was a comfort that has stayed with me all day.

At 5:52 am this morning I was started awake by the sound of someone knocking rhythmically somewhere in my house. It seemed to be in the bedroom. My heart was beating rapidly as my eyes scanned the still dark room for a sign of anyone who could be present. I heard a cat sneeze and immediately assumed that the noise I had heard was the sound of a cat heel banging off the hardwood floor as he scratched behind his ear. (I have heard this before.)

In the seconds it took me to come to this conclusion, my hand had gone to my belly, searching for the Cub. Mama protection starts early. He was moving. I could feel him kicking my hand. He kicked me several times before getting quiet.

I smiled and snuggled up next to my husband, happy that my Cub was fine. As I drifted off to sleep, I realized that perhaps the knocking noise was my own mind waking me up to feel the Cub move. I went to bed last night worried that something was wrong because he hadn't been as active yesterday as he had been recently...and because a friend of mind's sister just lost her baby.

In the end, the source of the knocking doesn't matter. All that matters is that the Cub is fine. He is healthy and moving and growing bigger everyday. Just 16 days until I see him again. Until then, I hope he keeps on rapping to let me know he's wonderful.

Pain, Pain Go Away

January 12, 2011 at 6:40 pm

AT 2:45 AM, I woke to the sound of our doorbell ringing, or what I thought was our doorbell ringing. I awoke completely and found the Cub kick, kick, kicking away. I thought, "Wow, he knocks and he rings the doorbell!" Pretty talented for a 24 week old fetus.

And then later in the day, the pain started. Severe, sharp stabbing pain in my lower abdomen and pelvis. I am almost positive that it is IBS. My stomach was cramping, too. I still have shooting pains in my pelvic region and my belly button area feels heavy. I am resisting the urge to call my doctor, simply because I am so sure it is bowel related. But I am scared nonetheless.

I drank several glasses of water and took a nap. Now, I am back up again working and trying to take my mind off of it.

Allegedly, the Cub is two days from viability, but I know that if he came now the outcome would not be all that good.

Stay with me Cub, please.

Calling the Doctor

January 12, 2011 at 10:12 pm

THE PAIN CAME BACK. I have a call into my doctors. Will update when I can.

Just 13 weeks to go. Hold tight, my Cub.

Safe and Sound

January 13, 2011 at 5:05 am

I ARRIVED IN PITTSBURGH at around 11:30 pm. By 3 am, I was being released with a dual diagnosis: ruptured ovarian cyst and round ligament pain. I remain in pain, but the Cub is perfect, and there are no signs of pre-term labor.

The sharp stabbing pain turned severe right around 9:30 or so. My doctor said to come up to obstetric triage immediately. By the time I hit the halfway point (Washington, PA), the snow had started.

They checked me in and strapped a monitor to my Cub spot, and we could hear is heart hammering away in there. He kicked the doppler several times, even knocking it off twice. There is no doubt that my boy is a healthy kid.

My blood pressure was great, but my pulse was elevated. (Really?!?!) Everything else was fine. No blood or protein in my urine. My cervix was closed and long. I had no contractions.

After about three hours, my team of doctors (the Cub and I get a whole team!) decided that it was an ovarian cyst rupture and round ligament pain that was causing all of the pain. I certainly hope they are right because I remain in pain still.

As relieved as I am, it was difficult for me. I had to recite my obstetric history five times, and since you all know that it involves infant murder, placenta abruption and newborn death, and other scary things, you will appreciate the additional pain it caused me to repeat all of that.

In addition, I kept thinking that I was at this stage of pregnancy—just about 24 weeks—when Nicholas was born. I know this baby is strong, but his chance of surviving outside of me right now are so slim.

In the long, difficult wait between doctor's examines and blood work, I was lulled into peacefulness by the rhythmic thumping of the Cub's heartbeat. It was like a lullaby. I kept telling him how much I loved him and that we could make it until he's ready.

Once we were let go, I made my way through the darkened hallways and stopped at the stairwell stunned. It had snowed another two inches while I was in triage. I took a deep breath and slowly made my way to my car. I slid from the hospital to the Fort Pitt Bridge and slipped my way through Washington and on into Wheeling.

We are home now. I am still in pain, but as my team assured me—this is no threat to the baby. The pregnancy is strong. The baby is good. Now up to bed we go. I owe my son a story, and my kitties some snuggles.

There Are Some Things You Just Can't Shake

January 14, 2011

It started the other day when I was roaming through the bookstore, my regular pastime. I stumbled onto a section of infertility books, and I caught my breath, remembering the many years of sad, sad months I spent reading every book I could find on how to get pregnant. Although those years are behind me now there's a cub hanging out in my belly, the trauma of those decades (yes, just about two decades of trying) still linger.

Later in the day, I was listening to the radio and heard a woman talking about her quest to have a child. I heard the heartbreak in her voice, and it took me right back to where I was six months ago. In some ways, it seems like a lifetime ago. In other ways, it seems like just yesterday.

Last night, I was looking for something in my bathroom closet and I found my stash of fertility monitor test strips and pregnancy tests. I took the bag off the shelf and cried. So many cycles of waiting for that second line.

I am not living in the past, but trying to move on. I am no longer in agony every month when my period comes to prove once again that I am not going to be a mother. Instead, the Cub is growing big and strong inside me. He will be here so soon.

Today, we are 24 weeks. Just 13 weeks to go and this Cub is all mine. Cannot wait to see that lovely face.

We Started on the Nursery!

January 15, 2011

I PUT MY FEARS aside and went with Jim to pick out our wallpaper and paint for the nursery today.

We chose a lovely tree print wallpaper for the top, a white chair rail, and lemon verbena (a sagey green) for the bottom. It is all washable and super durable. It should be done in about three weeks. I am so excited! After it is done, we will order and put together his furniture. He won't sleep in there until he is six months old, but all of his things will be in there.

He has quite a pile of belongings, certainly more than I had when I was still a fetus. (No, I don't have fetus envy. LOL.) I can't wait to see him wearing his little duds.

I know that there may be scary days ahead in this pregnancy, but I have to keep my faith that he is well.

I got a call today from my doctor saying I have a very mild urinary tract infection. She said she wouldn't even treat it if I wasn't pregnant, but UTIs can get very bad quickly in pregnancy and can lead to pre-term labor. She gave me an antibiotic, and I started it today.

In other news, I am working on a registry and getting lots of advice from friends (thank you Missy, Angie, and Lisa!) on what I need to get my world ready for my little boy. Some days, like right this minute, I feel overwhelmed by the voice in my heart shouting, "I'm going to be a Mom!"

Back to Work

January 18, 2011

I GO BACK into the classroom tomorrow. It will be hard. I have worked quite a bit over the break, but it's all been from my comfy chair and home office. Now, I will spend several hours on my feet every day, including walking all over campus. We'll get through it!

In fact, my doctor is glad I am working. Otherwise, he said, I would worry too much with all that time on my hands. I wonder....

In any case, I am trying to ensure I take enough healthy snacks not to get tired. I am loading up my car with bottles of water, too. I need to stay hydrated. I am glad I have a good parking spot now. I only have to walk 50 feet to get into my classroom building. Usually, I have to walk at least a mile.

I am wondering about how my colleagues (most of them do not know) will react to my big baby belly. It's rare to see a pregnant woman on campus, so I am sure I will stand out.

The Cub and I will make it, though. I am sure of that.

We had a good moment today. Cub's car seat and stroller arrived, and Jim came home for a layover and brought them in the house for me. I think it really touched him to see more things for Cub. I had pulled my shirt up over my belly and asked him if I looked bigger to him, and he caressed my Cub spot and said, "Yes. You really are." I almost cried.

It's the little moments that mean the most.

What's in a Name?

January 21, 2011

I HAVE BEEN CALLING the Cub "the Cub" for quite a long time. I mean, his Dad has always reminded me of a lion, so it just seemed obvious that his offspring would be a lion cub. Increasingly, however, I find myself referring to him in my head as Nicholas, my other son's name.

I am not sure where this is coming from. I guess maybe because every time I say the words "my son," they are always followed by the name "Nicholas." I know the Cub is not Nicholas, so it is almost surprising when I hear my inner voice call him that.

Maybe if we were already calling him by his actual name (which could be James or Tristan), then it wouldn't happen. But I am guessing I will probably still call the boy Cub for a long time after he is born, which is just fine with me! Maybe that could be his official name, Cub Greer. Hehehehe.

We are now at the 25 week point. As I type this, Cub is kicking me like crazy, and I am loving every second of it. He now has some cloth diapers (have to post pics of those later...so cute), a car seat and stroller, clothes, some toys, and some other odds and ends. His room should be done in a couple of weeks. He will be here himself in 12 weeks.

Jim said this morning, while looking at my ever-increasing Cub spot (which is now more like a Cub parking lot) that he didn't think I would get this big. (Wait until the end!) I had told him that with Nicholas I lost about 27 lbs. Of course, I realize now that it wasn't just that I was overweight that made me lose weight (it's common with obese mothers), but it is further proof that Nicholas was a very sick baby for a very long time.

This pregnancy is much more like my first than my second. Thankfully, I have only gained about 11 pounds. (With Samantha I gained 100!) But other things about it are quite similar: the shape of my belly, the stretch marks (boo), and the movement. He is an active little guy just like my daughter. I wonder if he will get as big? She was 8 lbs. 12 oz. I guess since he is coming early, he will weigh a bit less.

There are days when I absolutely cannot wait to see that handsome little face. Today is one of them. The more I prepare our home for him, the more excited I get about his arrival.

See you in three months, Cub-o. xxoxoxoxoxoo

PTSD Is Not Just an Another Acronym

January 24, 2011

I THINK MANY PEOPLE doubt the effects of PTSD. While most people can understand the soldier's post-war post-traumatic stress (shell shock when I was a kid), few people I have talked to truly understand PTSD caused by other traumas. I hope this entry stands as a statement for those of us who suffer from this devastating mind warp.

As I have written about previously, my house burned down in 2004. My cats were killed in the blaze, and I lost everything else: family mementos, most of my son's possessions, all of my daughter's things, and all of my writing. To this day I remain fearful of fire whistles, thinking the truck is heading to my house again. The fire also made me paranoid about everyday activities that would not frighten others, like leaving Christmas lights plugged in all night.

But those types of worries are to be expected from a person who has suffered a loss. PTSD is different in that it takes a seemingly benign situation and turns it into irrational fear. Tonight provides an excellent example.

Around 4 pm this evening, I realize my furnace didn't seem to be working. I looked at it, but I had no idea what I was seeing. After a few calls to the husband, his family, and some friends, I realized I had to call an HVAC guy. Meanwhile, I began to panic.

The house is going to burn down. This is just the way it happened before. The furnace ran and ran and ran, but it wasn't working well. The house stayed cold, no matter how long the furnace was on. My kitties are going to die. I am going to lose everything.

Overreacting? Of course. Able to be helped? Not by my own will.

I began to have flashbacks. Flames. Kitties dying in agony. The windows bursting from the heat. The sidewalk slick with fire hose ice.

Before long I was overcome with fear and crying, holding both cats on my lap in sheer terror.

The phone rang. Jim was calling to find out if the furnace had been repaired. He gently coaxed me back to rationality. By the time the repairman was finished, I was stable again. I calmly asked the repairman about the probability of fire. He explained it was extremely unlikely given my furnace's multitude of safety features. I was able to believe him.

PTSD is a serious syndrome. It never goes away completely. It can only be managed, which is why I have asked my doctors to have a psychologist on duty the day my son is born. Even if all goes well (which is the expectation), there is still a good chance that I will experience PTSD right there in the operating room with flashbacks to the night Nicholas was born. The only way to diminish the damage is to be prepared and to share my experiences.

I live in the shadow of PTSD, but I will not let it pull me into the darkness forever.

The Cub Has Big Eyes!
January 25, 2011

WELL, I DON'T really think they are bigger than any other 25 week old fetus eyes, but they were staring right at me today at the ultrasound. It was amazing. I got to see his cute little lips, too. And his heart is perfect, beating strong. The rest of the appointment was equally excellent.

He's up to a buff 2 lbs. and in the 62nd percentile for fetuses his age. His head is still dating a week in advance of his age (of course, he has MY brains!) and he starting to look like a human baby.

When the tech found his cute little self, I said, "Hey, I know that baby!" He kicked me. I embarrassed him already, I guess.

Then, I went to see my ob. All is great with me. My glucose tolerance test came back normal, so no gestational diabetes. My blood pressure was normal (113/78). No protein in my urine. They did find a bit of evidence that I might still have the UTI, but it could just be left over from the infection.

I now have to see my doctors every two weeks. We will set a C-section date in one month. At that time, I will have another ultrasound to assess his growth.

He'll be here in 11 weeks. Just 11 weeks!

When I saw that Cubby face today, I felt overcome with so many emotions. Every day that goes by, it gets more real. As soon as I saw him today, I started thinking of him as Tristan. It looks like that might be his name.

I wanted so much to hug him, but all I could do is pat my belly and wait for him to kick me back. I hope he knows how much I already love him.

Sharing MY Son

January 30, 2011

YOU CAN IMAGINE that I am fiercely protective of Cub, but I can share him...a little.

I try to encourage Jim to experience as much of the Cub as possible. I mean, he can never experience the Cub like I can, but I put his hand on my big Cub belly and hope the Cub moves. He gives up after a few seconds, though. And the Cub is a wily kind of baby, so as soon as you try to feel him, he stops kicking.

Today, he finally felt the Cub kick, a joy I have experienced several times a day since Christmas Eve. I kept telling him he was missing out because I giggle every single time. It never gets old. We were watching a movie, and I moved his hand over where the Cub was kicking. A few seconds later, the Cub kicked him right in the elbow.

I wish he was more excited about interacting with Cub, but I understand it is hard for him. I live with the Cub every minute of every day, and wow, do I feel lucky to be able to do so.

I am not going to miss this pregnancy. The fear of something going wrong has hung over it like a tall shadow. I will miss those kicks, though, and that my son is with me always.

10 weeks, 4 days until his blessed person arrives.

February 2011

Interrogating Memory, Searching for Truth

February 8, 2011

ALL THIS TERM my students and I have been discussing the reliability of memory. Most of us are sure events happened just as we remembered them, but time and time again, we discover that other people present have far different recollections. Who's wrong? Who's right? Can we ever know what really happened? Leaving Truth up to the veracity of our memories can have unintended consequences, as I discovered at the Cub doctor today.

I have told the story of my son Nicholas' birth here many times. He was born prematurely due to complete placenta previa and an abruption. I lost nearly half of my blood supply, and later, I would lose him. He died after living one week. Those are the facts. All the other details–the sound the nurses' shoes made while they were walking in my blood, my last thoughts before they wheeled me into surgery, the way my son looked while we waited for his helicopter to arrive to take him to Children's Hospital–are subjective and difficult, if not impossible, to prove.

On the other hand, the type of C-section cut should be easy to remember, but perception, especially in times of great trauma, can color even the most factual parts of an experience.

I learned today that the cut the doctor made when he removed Nicholas was not a classical C-section incision (vertical) but a lower uterine segment C-section (transverse or horizontal). Knowing this changes everything about the rest of this pregnancy and labor.

After reviewing the records, it has become clear I got confused about what I remembered because of the trauma of the situation. I remember my doctor apologizing to me for having to make the vertical cut. I have believed for almost a decade that he said those words AFTER the surgery, but he actually said them BEFORE. All of this data, including our conversation, is in the records.

How could it have been missed? How could I have been mistaken?

It did take the doctor's office until just last week to send the files to my current doctor's office, even though we requested them at six weeks. (21 weeks for paperwork to arrive!?!?!)

As my doctor explained her findings in my records, I immediately knew what it meant: I can VBAC. I can have my baby naturally. I became so excited I jumped off the exam table (sans pants) and hugged my doctor. I was so thrilled, not just about being able to labor naturally, but about being mostly out of risk for uterine rupture. My risk of my uterus tearing during VBAC is now less than 1%. When we thought I had a classical C, it was 90%+.

I still worry about pre-term labor. (It's a possibility for all pregnant women.) But now I know that if it should happen that my son and I have a much higher chance of surviving it.

I intend to have a birth much like that with my daughter: unmedicated and unaided until the last minute. They will monitor my son's status during labor, and hopefully, all will be well, like it was with Samantha. She was born in four hours and weighed a healthy 8 lbs. 12 oz. (I have verified these details with other people, and have seen her medical records.)

Not only is natural birth healthier for me and will give me a shorter recovery time, but it is healthier and less risky for Cub.

Of course, all this means that Cub probably won't arrive until two more weeks than when we expected. (Probably closer to his due date.) And he could go over that. Samantha was two weeks late. It also means, it would make it harder for Jim to be around for the birth, given that his job takes him out of the area several times a week.

But in the end, I know that this is what is best for me and Cub.

For the first time in a decade, I feel unafraid of pregnancy and delivery. I lived with the specter of Nicholas' birth and what I thought were lifelong problems with pregnancy and childbirth. Suddenly, I find myself in the normal risk category, and I am still in shock.

There is a chance that we will have to deliver via C-section in the end, but it is nowhere near the 100% chance I had when I got up this morning. Just like that, life can change. This time, it was for the better.

Researching Natural Childbirth Options

February 10, 2011

I NEVER, ever could have imagined I would be sitting here at my desk researching the best possibilities for a successful, unmedicated, natural childbirth. The whole idea of the Cub coming out on his own instead of out the escape hatch wasn't even on my list of remote possibilities just two days ago, but here I am doing what I do best: learning.

My daughter's birth was beautiful. My water broke at noon, contractions began at 2 pm, and at 6:02 pm, Samantha Christine was staring out at the world. Yes, it hurt. It hurt very, very badly, but I will do it again in a second. I had no drugs, no preparation, and no real support. (Her father was a tool to put it nicely.) In any case, I do want to be a little more prepared this time, and so I am considering just which method to choose.

Given I already practice meditation and yoga, I am leaning towards hypnobirthing. It is a pioneering and scientifically backed method that helps women go through the pains of childbirth with relative ease. It's basically a relaxation method to help women roll with the worst labor has to offer. Also known as the Mongan Method, hypnobirthing helps women get in a zone and become one with her body and baby during labor and delivery. This method sounds like it was made for me.

I have yet to check out Lamaze or the Bradley method. I can't do water birth because the Cub must be monitored at all times given the previous C-section, or I would most definitely choose that route.

In any case, there is much to be done before he decides to make his appearance. Is it even possible to love this baby more than I did just the other day? Wish I could hug you, Cub.

Is This Your First?

February 15, 2011

I ABSOLUTELY DETEST this question. When a stranger asks if the baby I am carrying is my first child, I have a choice. I can say no and answer the questions that are sure to follow, or I can say yes and feel like I am negating the existence of Samantha and Nicholas. But when an obstetrician asks, I have no choice but to say, "This is my fifth pregnancy. Two live births. No living children." Most good OBs will leave it at that, but nurses are sometimes more intrusive.

I felt completely exhausted after I got home from work and took a nap. When I got up, I went to the bathroom and notice three little pink spots on the toilet tissue. I freaked out! (Remember all that spotting throughout the first trimester!?) I looked again and there was no more. I decided that it was related to a rough bowel movement I had earlier in the day and TRIED to pass it off as nothing.

For the next four hours, I obsessively checked for more spots, but the TP came back clear every single time. I debated on calling my doctor, just to ease my mind, but I figured that would result in another dark and lonely, one-hour drive to the hospital.

I went to bed and read to Cub like always, but could not sleep. Not long after my head hit the pillow, I felt a heaviness in my pelvic area that would not go away. At 1:20 am, I broke down and called my doctor.

I was surprised when the doctor on call didn't seem worried, but she did strongly urge me to come in right away just to ease my mind. Given that on this day in my last pregnancy, my son was born, I needed some piece of mind.

Off we went in the middle of the night alone. Jim is on the road.

After several hours of monitoring, we learned all is well. No signs of pre-term labor, no blood found anywhere, and no positive answer on the spotting. They think it is from a small rectal tear. (Yay me!)

The best part, of course, was hearing Cub's heartbeat and then seeing him on the big screen. Lovely, lovely Cub all safe and cozy.

Unfortunately, a nurse took down my information and when we arrived at the detested question, I gave my pat answer. She then asked what happened to my children. I told her that Nicholas was born early and that Samantha was murdered. She asked, "Who would ever want to hurt your child?" And I briefly explained the story. She asked more questions. I refused to answer. As I have said before, Samantha is my daughter. She had a life. That life should be respected and honored, not seen as a spectacle. Our lives are not an episode of trash TV.

We were discharged at 5:45 a.m. Thankfully, my friend Kristy was praying for us. I fell asleep at the wheel and woke up going 75 miles an hour down a steep grade just as my car left the blacktop and hit the grass. I quickly pulled her back on the road. We were scared but not hurt.

Cub has been on many adventures and so far, we are both well. Hopefully, our good fortune will hold until he arrives, strong and handsome. He's not my first, but he may be my only living and breathing child.

Daycare and Hypnobirthing

February 16, 2011

CUB NOW HAS a daycare for when I go back to work in the fall. It is on campus, just a few buildings away from my office. It seems nice, and the price is very good. It will be hard to leave him there each day, but I know at any point I can dash in to see him. (You know I will.)

It seemed a bit strange to be talking about him in such a concrete way. I mean, I do that in writing all the time, but to actually sign him up for something made him even more real to me. We are almost at 29 weeks, which means that his chances of survival if he was born early continue to climb. We are around 85% now.

I have been doing research on childbirth methods. Even though my birth with my daughter was a good one, I know it could be less chaotic and less painful if I understand it more. I just finished reading *Ina May's Guide to Childbirth*. It was excellent. I learned much from her wisdom and wish that she could attend Cub's birth. However, it would not be safe to have him at home (aargh!) because of the previous C-section. Off to the hospital we will go.

In any case, it looks like we will do hypnobirthing. Yeah, that's right. I am mostly a hippie at heart. I researched all of the methods, and it makes the most sense given I already practice yoga and meditation. Basically, hypnobirthing involves controlled breathing and deep relaxation. And, with a good chance I will be laboring alone (for part or all of the birth), it is good for that, too.

Clarifications

February 17, 2011

I FINALLY heard from the doctor that delivered Nicholas, and what he told me was excellent vis-a-vis my upcoming attempt at natural birth.

According to Ina May Gaskin (and other fine researchers/practitioners) the rate of success with VBAC (vaginal birth after a C-section) is limited by several factors:

1. the type of incision (vertical or horizontal)
2. the type of suture (single or double)
3. the size of the baby

It turns out that I score high on the first two. The incision was a horizontal incision. No, you cannot always tell from your scar how they cut your uterus, but the doctor confirmed that the records were right: my incision is horizontal, which means that my chances of uterine abruption during an attempt at vaginal delivery are very low.

The other potential complication I faced was the time of suture. Single sutures, which became commonplace around the time insurance companies became so powerful, have been known to rupture during vaginal labor attempts. Thankfully, my doctor sewed me up twice, which is the best possible suture.

As for the big baby issue. It MIGHT be an issue, but not likely, given that my daughter was 8 lbs 12 oz.

I am getting more excited every single day. 29 weeks pregnant now. He should be here in 10-12 weeks or less. (I wonder if he's like a pizza...if he doesn't get here on time, he's free?!?! LOL).

I cannot wait to see him. During a meeting today, he was kicking me hard and other people could see him moving. That's the first time I have shared him with someone other than Jim. It was wonderful.

Co-Sleeping

February 20, 2011

ALTHOUGH OUR NURSERY walls are not yet finished, we managed to clean out the room so it is ready to go. We also bought Cub his co-sleeper bed yesterday, so he will have a place to sleep when he gets home. Of course, we had to take it down to avoid cat-tamination, but it's cute and should be a cozy bed for Cub.

I had intended on co-sleeping with him from the beginning, but I wasn't sure how Jim would feel about it. After he saw the little bed I picked he seemed much more in favor of it. Then, I had him read Dr. Sears' advice on co-sleeping, and he was even more convinced that it was best for me and Cub.

Although Dr. Sears strongly advocates for in-bed, co-sleeping because it might actually prevent Sudden Infant Death Syndrome (SIDS) because mom and baby are more in tune with one another, I just don't feel comfortable with it for long periods of time. I fully expected in-bed naps with Cub, and of course, in-bed breastfeeding, but I think I would be too scared of him sleeping in bed with me and Jim. What if the blanket fell on his face or a pillow or something horrible like that?

All that said, I know of many moms who bed share with babies, and they are just fine. Perhaps I will wait and see how it goes.

One thing is for sure, the cats will be jealous of this little bed. I would be, too!

Breech Baby, Breech Baby, Turn Your Butt Around

February 24, 2011

I HAD A GREAT appointment today. It began with an ultrasound and ended with a regular OB appointment. Everything looks good–all but the Cub is now breech.

When we checked in on him today, he was lying across my tummy with his butt down and his feet and legs over his head. Up until this point, he has been a good baby with his head down ready to greet the world. I will be 30 weeks tomorrow, so I have many weeks left for him to get back into his birth position. Cross your fingers for us. It would be an annoying turn of events if after finding out I can VBAC, I end up needing to have a C-section because he is breech.

Other than that, Cub is super awesome! He weighs 3 lbs. 8 oz., which means he is in the 65th percentile for his gestational age. All his parts looked healthy and stronger. And he has hair! Little tufts of hair right above his ears.

The best part of the exam was when he was playing with his little Cub feet. Eventually, he stuck his big toe in his mouth and sucked on it. At least I know what he is doing in there when I feel him thumping around.

I fully expected him to hold up a sign that said, "Please no more PB&J sandwiches." Instead, he was having a very good time in there. At one point, he turned and faced me, and I burst into tears. He is so handsome!

The tech turned on the 3D, but he would not cooperate enough to let us take his pic. I did see him very clearly, though, which was both cool and creepy. I so wanted to snuggle with him and kiss him all over. But he is still growing in there, so I will let him do his job.

Meanwhile, I have been doing my job. My blood pressure and all the other measurables are excellent. No signs of pre-eclampsia or any other condition. I hope things stay that way. It won't be long now. They told me to pack my hospital bag. At my next appointment, we will go over my birth plan. I will share a draft of it here in the coming days. Hooray for healthy Cub!

Birth Plan, Rough Draft
February 25, 2011

I HAVE STARTED on my birth plan. I will share it with my doctors in two weeks. Birth plans are more like wish lists, but it helps give me a blueprint for talking about the birth with my team.

Labor

- I would like to be free to walk around during labor.
- I wish to be able to move around and change positions at will throughout labor.
- I wish to be able to labor in water, if possible, throughout labor.
- For comfort, I wish to wear my own clothing during labor.
- I would like to eat and drink normally through labor and I will make easily digestible food choices.
- I would like the environment to be kept as quiet as possible with dim lighting.
- I would prefer to keep the number of vaginal exams to a minimum to reduce the possibility of infection.
- I prefer a hep lock to an iv unless medically necessary.

Monitoring

- I do not wish to have continuous fetal monitoring.
- While being monitored intermittently, I would like to have the option of having the monitor held by a nurse or my labor support people if the straps begin to bother me.

Labor Augmentation/Induction

- I do not wish to have the amniotic membrane ruptured artificially.
- I would prefer to be allowed to try changing position and other natural methods such as walking, nipple stimulation before Pitocin is administered if labor augmentation is necessary.
- I do not want to be induced.

Anesthesia/Pain Medication
- I am not interested in any pain medications.

Cesarean
- Unless absolutely necessary, I would like to avoid a Cesarean.
- If a Cesarean delivery is indicated, I would like to be fully informed and to participate in the decision-making process.
- I do not wish my labor support persons to be removed from the room during any surgical preparation.
- I do not consent to having my arms or hands strapped down unless I am unable to control them. I understand the necessity of maintaining a sterile surgical field.
- I wish my labor support person to take pictures and/or video tape the delivery.
- If the baby is not in distress, I wish the baby to be given to my labor support person or me immediately after birth.
- I do not wish the baby to be separated from me unless he is in distress. If the baby must be taken away, the father will accompany him.
- I would appreciate being allowed to breastfeed as soon as possible after birth, preferably in the recovery room.

Episiotomy
- I would prefer to tear than have an episiotomy, but welcome the use of compresses, massage, and positioning to prevent tearing.

Delivery
- I would like to be allowed to choose the position in which I give birth, including squatting.
- I would appreciate not being held to stringent time limits and avoiding any interventions like vacuum extraction and forceps for as long and the baby and I are doing well.
- Please allow Spontaneous Bearing Down and refrain from

any loud counting or yelling to "push", I would really like the chance to listen to and work with my body.
- I would appreciate having the room lights turned low for the actual delivery.
- I would appreciate having the room as quiet as possible when the baby is born.
- I would like to have the baby placed on my stomach/chest immediately after delivery.

Immediately After Delivery
- I would like my husband to cut the cord.
- I would prefer that the umbilical cord stop pulsating before it is cut. I would like to hold the baby while I deliver the placenta and any tissue repairs are made. I would like to hold the baby for at least fifteen minutes before he is photographed, examined, etc.
- I would like to have the baby evaluated and bathed in my presence.
- I plan to keep the baby near me following birth and would appreciate if the evaluation of the baby can be done with the baby on my abdomen, with both of us covered by a warm blanket, unless there is an unusual situation.
- If the baby must be taken from me to receive medical treatment, my husband or some other person I will designate will accompany the baby at all times.
- I would prefer to hold the baby rather than have him placed under heat lamps.
- I do not want a routine injection of Pitocin after the delivery to aid in expelling the placenta.

Postpartum
- I would like a private room, if available.
- I do not wish to be separated from my baby at any time.

Breastfeeding
- I plan to breastfeed and would like to begin nursing very

shortly after birth.
- I do not want the baby to be given a pacifier or any artificial nipples.
- I do not consent to any supplementation with either formula or glucose water. If supplementation is medically necessary it should be discussed with me beforehand and be done with expressed breast milk if possible and through a supplemental feeding system (finger feeding with the aid of a tube or cup feeding) as opposed to a bottle.

March 2011

Moving Right Along

March 3, 2011

MY CUB CHORES are slowly getting accomplished, but I still have so much left to do before his beautiful self makes his arrival.

The walls in his room have been painted and wallpapered. He has a bassinet and a Pack-n-Play. He has a bunch of clothes. And I take a tour of the maternity ward soon.

He still needs more cloth diapers and his crib and furniture, but I have a bit of time to get that done over spring break week.

He scares me sometimes because he doesn't move as much as usual, but then a few hours later, he is back to his rambunctious self.

As soon as the nursery is done, I will post pics. It probably will not be for 10 days or so. I can't wait until that part of my list is checked off.

We are at 31 weeks here in a few hours. Not too far left to go. Just nine weeks until his due date.

I'm All for Believing

March 10, 2011

I RIPPED OFF this title from a Missy Higgins song. In it she implores,

> Pull back the shield between us, and I'll kiss you.
> Drop your defenses, and come into my arms.
> I'm all for believing. I'm all for believing.

She is talking about a romantic relationship here, but today it entered my head on my way home for the Cub doctor. I am all for believing I really might bring Cub home safe and sound.

I know many people take parenthood for granted (and even begrudge it a little). I know I did when I was 17 and completely clueless. Before my innocence was totally lost when Samantha was murdered. Somehow, though, I managed to overcome the fear of child loss when I became pregnant with Nicholas. Even though it was clear the pregnancy was in trouble from the start, I never, ever imagined he would not survive. Even when I began bleeding, I believed he would be fine, and I would bring his little bow-legged self home with me.

I was wrong.

The two early losses that followed ended any kind of naiveté I ever had about pregnancy and motherhood. I believed after that fourth loss I would be lucky to survive a pregnancy, if I ever got pregnant again, and my children would probably not survive at all.

This pregnancy has been scary at times, but each day Cub grows gives me hope I will be a mother...and soon. I remain, of course, somewhat skeptical, but today's appointment added another check in the positive column that has been edging ever closer to completion since that August night I found out I was pregnant.

My favorite doctor was working today, and I was thrilled to see him. He is way smarter than I am (a rare find in a doctor), and he is really funny. He can quote statistics and other facts like no other doctor I have seen, and he has practical experience to go with all his "book learnin'."

He said to keep doing what I am doing. All is well with me and with Cub. Cub is a little bit big (65%), but not too big, and he should weigh in at about 7 lbs. or a little over at full-term.

I asked about the cramps and other pains I had been having this week, and he said not to worry, they were just Braxton Hicks contractions down low. He said they are normal.

I asked if I went into pre-term labor today if Cub could be born vaginally. He said, "Yes. You made it!"

I stopped talking for a second (that's hard for me to do), and asked him to repeat himself. He said, "You made it! If he was born now, he would have the same survival odds as a full-term infant: 98%."

I said nothing, but I could feel my heart racing.

We then talked about the birth and the possibility of an emergency C-section if Cub went into distress. He said, "Don't worry. If that happens, we have a team of experts on staff 24/7 who can have you in the OR and prepped in five minutes or less. We will save you and him."

I sighed.

We finished up the visit by listening to Cub's heartbeat: a healthy 130 bpm and by measuring my fundal (uterine) height. I am measuring at 4 weeks over my actual size because of the extra me-ness. (Okay, abdominal fat.) Everything is good: blood pressure, blood sugar, iron, and all that stuff.

As I was walking out, he said to me: "You just have 36 more days until he is full-term. If you can make it, then there is nothing at all to be afraid of. It is even shorter than Lent. 36 days, Christina."

I left there with Missy Higgins' song in my head. I AM all for believing ... that labor will go well, Cub will come home safe and sound, and in the end, I will get to raise my beautiful son.

Thanks for believing, especially in the moments when I just couldn't.

Third Trimester, Same as the First

March 15, 2011

AND IT FINALLY KICKED IN: the third trimester. I am exhausted, nauseated, bloated, achy, and just plain wore out. We only have 32 days to go until Cub is full-term, though, so the countdown is really taking off now.

I am still working full-time and really feel for women the world over who must do hard labor while pregnant. I can't imagine how they do it. I am so tired all the time now I just want to sleep, but work goes and so do Cub and I.

He is having a lazy day in there, waking up only after breakfast and lunch. I envy his womb comforts.

His room is just about entirely finished...just in time for the shower this weekend. I can't wait to see my friends and to show off my belly bump. I have been neglecting my friends this semester so it will be nice to just spend some time with all of them.

Now I no longer have to worry so much about Cub dying if he is born early (anything can happen), my fears have switched to stillborn and birth defects that weren't caught on ultrasound. It doesn't help that a woman in my group just had a stillborn baby and another one just found out her son has a hole in his heart. I don't dwell on these fears, but they float in the back of my head when I can't sleep at night.

I am so incredibly excited about Cub's upcoming arrival. Time has gone so slowly this pregnancy. I just can't wait to finally hold him.

Just a Sprinkle a Day...

March 23, 2011

SOMETIMES I JUST can't resist bad puns for titles. Thanks for reading anyway.

I am home from work today because I had a lot of pains last night. Backache, menstrual-like cramping, and stomach cramps. After all that fun, I couldn't sleep, so rather than try to get through a work day and commute on an hour's rest, I stayed home to get more sleep and to get caught up on grading.

This past Saturday was Cub's baby shower, and it was so much fun. I missed my friends who could not attend, but was so grateful for the ones who could make it. We played games, ate cupcakes, and did girl stuff. What a wonderful way to spend a spring afternoon. Thanks to my girls, Lisa and Diane, for making it all happen.

Of course, as is typical of me, I took pics of the pre-shower and the after-shower, but forgot to take pics during the shower

Making it safely to the shower date was a major milestone for us. There were so many times I never thought we'd make it this far. We will be 34 weeks this Friday (just two more days), which means if he comes then or thereafter his chances of survival will be better than ever. He will be able to breathe on his own because his lungs will be developed.

I get to see him on ultrasound tomorrow, and I can't wait. I haven't seen him in nearly a month!

He almost has everything he needs. I have ordered his cloth diapers (and my MIL gave me some at the shower), and just about everything he needs. I still need to pick up a baby bathtub, a nursing cloth, a nursing pump, and a swing. Thanks again to my wonderful friends for helping me out.

Sleeping Cubs Don't Lie

March 24, 2011

I HAD A ROUTINE appointment today, which included an ultrasound, a non-stress test (NST), and an OB checkup. In the end, all was fine, but there were moments of sheer terror that have left me shaken and a little sad.

The ultrasound was first. We peaked in on a sleeping Cub. Even though I could see his heart beating, seeing him asleep like that was horrifying. He would not wake up. He has never slept through an ultrasound before, so the longer the scan went on, the more frightened I became. Then, when they recorded his heart rate it was low: just 118.

I started crying and begging for him to wake up. "Wake up, Cub, please. Please, wake up." But he slept on. At one point, the tech put the scanner over his face to get a profile, and I screamed. He looked like he was dead. He was so still. Within seconds the dead faces of my daughter and son morphed over Cub's. I panicked. Again, begging him to wake up for me. At one point, he moved his foot, but he never moved his head. I couldn't breathe.

The tech kept assuring me he was fine, just resting, but when she left the room to confirm the results with the radiologist, I started shaking, thinking that even if his heart was beating now, it would not be for long. The tech was gone for what seemed like much longer than usual. When she returned, she said everything was just fine. She said he weighs 5 lbs., 13 oz. and is in the 85th percentile for growth. Even this news did little to calm my fears.

I headed up to my OB appointment, and as soon as I walked in they set me up on the NST machine. It measures fetal heart rate and contractions. I freaked out more because I thought they had gotten bad news from the ultrasound tech and were double checking. It turns out that my doctors begin doing NSTs at every single appointment at 32 weeks on, so this was simply routine.

Two-Week Wait

They hooked him up to the monitor, and he was still sleeping. I must have looked scared because they came back in and shocked him with these two zappers. He woke up then! His heart rate was totally normal, and they kept reassuring me he was fine. In addition to the good heart rate scan, they also said his other measurements were perfect: respiration, amniotic fluid, size.

Evidently, they figured I was going to keep freaking out because they said if it will make me feel better that I could come in in a week and get another NST. I took them up on their offer. From now on, I will be making the trip to Pittsburgh once a week. They will do another growth scan on ultrasound in two weeks as a routine procedure.

At one point, I told my doctor I was worried. And she said, "Of course, you are. You're his mother." And my heart swelled. Yes, I am his mother. He will come home with me soon. He will.

April 2011

It's Better to be Safe Than Sorry

April 5, 2011 at 3:21 pm

SORRY ABOUT THE CLICHED titled, but my cold-clogged head doesn't allow for much creativity at the moment. I am behind on entries, so I figured I should take a few minutes to catch up.

Last week was a big week. I went to a new therapist to discuss ways of avoiding or limiting post-partum depression after Cub is born. I like my new therapist. She seemed knowledgeable, friendly, and compassionate. As we talked, she continuously said, "Well, uh, you've had a colorful life" and "Wow, that's interesting." I still can't tell if surprising a therapist is a good thing or bad thing, but let's just say that she is right. My life has been anything but dull.

We set up a plan to work on getting ready for his arrival and another plan for after he gets here. With these plans in place, this blog, and everyone in my little world knowing that I am at risk for PPD, I feel quite a bit better about facing the future. I just want to be a happy new Mom and love Cub with all of my heart. The last thing I want is for our first year together to be clouded by sadness and confusion.

Of course, just two days after I met with my new therapist I had an anxiety attack. I realize now what I was feeling was the beginning of this terrible cold that I still have, but at the time, I couldn't stop thinking that I was developing pre-eclampsia, which can be deadly for Mom and baby. I had all of the symptoms, which are the same symptoms for panic attacks and migraine headaches. (I have both!)

I showed up at my doctor's office already worried. They did a Non-stress Test (NST) like normal, and it went just fine, but when I explained my recent symptoms to my doctors, they sent me to L&D. I had a "trace" amounts of protein in my urine, but my BP was normal: 120/70, as it has been for the entire pg.

But they were concerned because I was concerned, so at L&D, they put a cuff on me and took my BP every 15 minutes. Again, it was totally normal. They also monitored Cub, who was "doing spectacular."

After five hours, they diagnosed me with migraines and GERD.

Meanwhile, because of the trace protein, they gave me a 24-hour urine kit to take home. Every single time I pee, I have to catch it in a hat, pour it into a container, and refrigerate it. Fun stuff, that. I am halfway done.

Anyway, I am terribly relieved that it's NOT pre-e. Of course, anything can happen, but I will see them in two days (and Cub, too).

They kept telling me, especially after I burst into tears, that if he came now, he would be fine.

Going Pony Shopping Soon

April 7, 2011

I HAD MY WEEKLY Cub appointment today. All went well in the end. I was even having little contractions, although I could not feel them.

I had a very scary moment when I first got there and they could not find the heartbeat for the NST. It was horrifying. It took four nurses to find it. When they finally did, I was so relieved, but also angry because once again I was alone.

They then sent me to ultrasound, where I saw a gorgeous, giant Cub-o making a big fuss. His big head was down and ready for birth. I knew he had moved yesterday on my way home from work. I could feel him crumple up in a ball and move down. I had horrible pain in my pubic mound and walking became uncomfortable. Of course, now that he has turned, I have to go pony shopping. I promised him a pony if he turned.

In any case, I had a long talk with my doctor about what to expect, and he said it is easy from here on out. I guess he meant for him because I still have to go through delivery. I cannot wait. I know it may sound insane, but I really do look forward to laboring and giving birth to Cub.

After dropping off my 24-hour urine sample (that was really fun...), they told me all was normal. No signs whatsoever of preeclampsia. My doctor told me I was very healthy and can expect a good outcome.

Now we wait. He is due May 6, but he could come at any time. Everything is ready for him. His room, his cloth diapers, his co-sleeper. Just waiting on my little lion cub to show his handsome face.

Falling Down the Rabbit Hole

April 12, 2011

SOME SUFFERERS describe it as being like Alice's journey down the rabbit hole. That is, a seemingly endless plummet over which the person has no control. Although the beginning of depression seems that way to me often, I prefer to use a musical term to describe this sometimes rapid descent: glissando.

Back in my choir days, we were required to memorize music terminology. Although I hated it at the time, that education has paid off. I have found those words are often the only terms that adequately describe my state of mind. In this case, glissando, or the sliding from one pitch to another, is the perfect word to articulate my latest round of mental troubles: depression.

I know it is normal to be depressed at the end of pregnancy. Hormone fluctuations, anxiety over the child's birth, and a host of other factors contribute to a feeling of sadness. In my case, it happened on Tuesday of last week. At 12:45 p.m. I could feel my emotions slowly slide from happy to depressed in a short time period, and I knew I couldn't stop it from happening.

It has improved some, but I am still struggling with crying spontaneously. I have told my doctors, and they said it is normal. I am hoping a visit to my therapist next week will help lessen the effects and prevent it from getting worse.

I wish it was as simple as being able to "cheer up" or "look forward to the Cub," but given that the basis of this depression is mostly physiological, a change of attitude or focus will not make it go away. I hope it is temporary. Perhaps the next glissando will move me upwards instead of down into darkness.

Non-Stress Test, My A$$

April 14, 2011

I HAD MY WEEKLY appointment today, and once again, my boy was being obstinate. Although they found his heartbeat after a while, he was not reactive enough, so they sent me in for a bio-physical profile ultrasound, and there he was kicking and drinking amniotic fluid and having a good old time!! He was breathing and sucking his thumb and basically, living a very fun life for a fetus. I was so relieved!

Anyway, it took me three hours to get in for the ultrasound, and I basically freaked out (though quietly behind a good book) until then. I was trying so hard not to panic, but that is hard to do when the person you love most in all the world might be in trouble.

In other news, I have lost four lbs. (no big deal), my blood pressure was perfect (120/70), and....my cervix is open and I am 30% effaced! That means that I could go any time now. My doctor told me to make sure my bag is packed (it is!).

So, this kid is slowly making his way into the world, but it won't be soon enough for me.

After the ultrasound, I went back down to MFM and told them to throw away my pink and blue non-stress test bands because I WILL NOT do another NST. It's ultrasounds from here on out.

Cub and I at Full-Term

April 17, 2011

WE HAVE ARRIVED at 37 weeks, which means Cub is fully baked. He will spend the remaining time making more body fat and growing a bigger brain.

Tubby Cubby

April 19, 2011

I HAD MY WEEKLY doctor's appointment today and found out that Cub is a big boy indeed. He's weighing in at a hefty 8 lbs. 4 oz., which puts him in the 90th percentile. I am so grateful for a healthy son.

If he goes to term, he could get as big as 10 lbs., which obviously would be huge, but my doctor doesn't think we will make it. She thinks that Cub will be coming this week. When she checked today, my cervix was fully ripe, but I was still just 1 cm dilated and

30% effaced. She said, though, that a ripe cervix is the biggest indication of impending labor.

I have been having cramps since 6 a.m. but not active labor cramps. He is head down with his face facing my spine, so all we are waiting for is for him to say, "It's go time, Mama!" I still believe I am going to get my Easter baby.

So close to holding him forever.

A Bittersweet Countdown

April 20, 2011

As Cub's approach draws near, I have had a bit of time to reflect on what it all means. I know I will not miss him living inside me. I have experienced that before, like so many other women, but the anxiety of this pregnancy has been so great I can't imagine it going on much longer. Nonetheless, I will miss the opportunity of being pregnant again. This is my last baby.

I have been pregnant five times. The first time was easy and wonderful. I felt great and enjoyed it. There were hard times because her father was not supportive, but my body loved being pregnant and it showed. My second pregnancy was miserable from the start. I was sick from the day of conception and nearly died giving birth. My two miscarriages were over before I knew what happened. And, of course, this Cub, oh, this wonderful, wonderful Cub. Despite the worry and that first trimester spotting, this has been an excellent pregnancy.

As the wind down begins, I can't help but mourn just a little for this chapter of my life, which is just about over. I won't miss the torture of trying to get pregnant, especially the fertility treatments. I won't miss the agony of waiting for a positive pregnancy test or the deep longing when I saw other Moms with their children.

I will miss the joy of being able to create a life. From the moment I met him, I wanted to have a child with Jim. I thought it would never happen after we broke up over and over again. But when I found we had finally achieved what had seemed impossible, I felt so much of my hopes and dreams had come true. Cub was created out of incredible love and will be raised in that soft, warm bubble.

I wish we were younger. We would give him a brother or sister. But Jim is against having another child, thinking it is best to concentrate on raising our boy. While one healthy child is more than a blessing, I hope that Cub won't be lonely.

With all of these mild pangs of sadness, there comes such incredible joy. Cub is a big, healthy boy! And this Mother's Day will be the first one in the history of me that I will have a living child.

I still believe he will make his appearance by this Easter, but even if that day comes and goes, he is still worth waiting for. After all, if I can wait 20 years, I can certainly wait a few more days. Of course, that doesn't mean I won't be sending him quiet vibes to encourage his appearance.

No Easter Cub

April 25, 2011

EASTER HAS COME and gone. No Cub. I don't mind waiting, but I sure could use a big Cub hug.

I was up all night with terrible pain. Either he is getting bigger, or he is getting closer to exiting. In any case, in he's in there.

We are 38 weeks 2 days, and he has 11 days to go until his official due date. The doctors keep saying any time now. I can wait. Really, I can.

I'm not 17 Anymore

April 25, 2011

As my due date approaches, things have gotten painful. My first pregnancy 20 years ago was nothing like this, but clearly, I am no longer 17.

With my first pregnancy I struggled with pain as my pelvic bones spread. I don't have that problem now, given that they are pretty much open at this point in my life.

In this pregnancy, I am experiencing a substantial amount of pain. Last night and for several hours today, I have had strong round ligament pain. Earlier tonight, I couldn't even walk it hurt so badly. I also have numbness in my right hand from carpal tunnel syndrome. And constant cramps. Needless to say, this part of pregnancy is not going so well.

Oh, and the hot flashes. I am so hot all of the time. I need a fan on everywhere I go. And headaches!

I know it is all worth it in the end, but right now, I just want to fall asleep and wake up to my snuggly Cub.

Making a Cub's Nest

April 27, 2011

I have been so tired over the past few weeks. I haven't been getting enough sleep because of the aches and pains, and I have felt sluggish and worthless. Today, however, I had a burst of energy, which could be seen as nesting.

Many people say pregnant women experience nesting throughout their pregnancy, but most report an increase in tending to their homes ready for their new babies at around five months or so. I hit a big period of that when we were putting the nursery together, and it really never came back.

Until today.

I have cleaned, washed, dried, scrubbed, buffed, and set up stuff for Cub. Although our second floor was all ready for Cub, our first floor was not. I will be spending quite a bit of time down here every single day, so getting his Fold'n'Go set up and his cloth diapers and wipes ready was really important. Thankfully, it's all done.

I have no idea what will happen at our appointment tomorrow, but I am guessing they will do a progress check and send me on my way. As long as Cub is fine, I guess that is the best I can hope for. I figure they will talk to me about induction, but I really have no interest in that. Even though I would love to see Cub right this very second, I know induction can be very painful and can lead to a C-section delivery. I want to avoid both.

In any case, my bag is packed and ready to go. I had to re-pack it after I found out Cub's size. There is little chance his big self will fit in newborn sizes. So I packed him some new clothes in 0-3 months.

The worst of the cramping has subsided, but I am still having trouble getting adequate rest because of pregnancy-induced carpal tunnel. But it really can't go on for much longer. If Cub doesn't come by 41 weeks (just two weeks away), then we will have to talk about induction.

Another Restless Night

April 30, 2011

CUB IS OFFICIALLY DUE in six days. I thought for sure he was coming last night because I had the worst contractions! They lasted for six hours, and then vanished.

I sure wish I was writing Cub's birth story. Instead, I am sitting at my table drinking water and trying to figure out the best place to go for a walk. At least I don't have to work today. I don't think I would make it.

May 2011

Another Scary Day

May 5, 2011

Yesterday was a long day, and I still have the headache to prove it. Cub was uncooperative again, and of course, it scared me.

I went to our usual weekly appointment to find that on the non-stress test, which I agreed to only so they could measure my contractions, Cub was unreactive. He had a normal heartbeat, but he wasn't moving around enough and had no heart accelerations as expected. It took them 15 minutes to find his heartbeat, but I knew Cub was alive in there because he had just been kicking me in the waiting room.

Nonetheless, they sent me to have an emergency ultrasound to confirm all was well. I could see Cub's heart beating nicely as soon as we began the scan, but he was sound asleep. (I had sugared up before going in, too.) The tech left the room to get a buzzer to zap him. Seconds after she walked out, I heard a woman scream.

At first, I couldn't tell if it was a cry or a laugh, but it became very clear within minutes that she was wailing. Seeing what I have seen, being where I have been, I knew she just found out her baby was dead.

I wanted to climb off the table and go to her, but what could I possibly say? Words are never more futile (and potentially painful) than after a child loss. I certainly couldn't tell her the truth; that the hole would never close. That even after the edges scarred, the wide, gaping cavern of loss would remain forever.

Instead, I tried sending her comforting thoughts, repeating "I'm sorry" over and over again.

When the tech returned with the buzzer, I asked her if the woman's baby was dead, and she nodded solemnly. I took a deep breath and focused on Cub again. After zapping his little butt, he began to move around like crazy. And what a giant Cub he has become. His hands look like newborn hands. I did not get to see his Cubby face, but the rest of him has filled out nicely since our last visit.

As I left ultrasound, I looked for the woman, whose face I felt certain I would recognize. She was now a member of a very sad club to which no one wishes to belong. She was nowhere in the halls. I hope they took good care of her.

My doctor, like always, says Cub could come any day now. I am still only 1 cm dilated, but my cervix is ultra-soft and now 50% effaced. He is due tomorrow, so....

I was still overwhelmed with sadness as I left the hospital. I felt the post-fear let down and tremendous sadness for the woman who just found out her baby had died inside her. I cried all the way home for both of us. I cried for her current loss and my previous ones, now woven together under a tapestry of joy known as Cub.

Guess Dates Come and Go

May 6, 2011

TODAY IS CUB'S due date or estimated date of delivery or guess date. Nope, he's not here yet. Still waiting.

It is getting harder just to exist. This pregnancy has been pretty easy physically until the last couple of weeks. I am in pain nearly every day and most nights. My doctor says it is normal for subsequent pregnancies, but it doesn't feel normal to me. Worst of all, it gets my hopes up.

Nonetheless, as I begin my 10th month of pregnancy I am grateful for the chance to carry Cub long enough so that he will be healthy. I am grateful that he exists at all.

Maybe he will come along on Mother's Day. What a present that would be!

Tristan's (Cub's) Birth Story

May 11, 2011

TRISTAN THOMAS "CUB" is now nearly a day old. It seems like a lifetime ago, though, when they brought him to my husband swaddled and needing a bottle. I have not slept in about 65 hours. I will sleep soon enough, but before I try once again to meet the sandman, I figured I would share the whole story of my son's birth.

On Monday, March 9, I walked out of the bathroom at 6:30 p.m. and my water broke. A big gush, just like on TV. I ran back to the bathroom and called Jim, who was fixing our hot water tank, which had just blown its water as well. I called my doctors, and they said to come in right away. We had to wait for my water to stop gushing and then off we went, stopping for a small snack on the way.

Tristan's (Cub's) Birth Story

By 8:34 I started having contractions. They were mild, but measurable. I couldn't wait to get to the hospital to find out if Cub was doing well and to see how much I had progressed towards birth. By the time they assessed me and Cub, it was 10:30 pm. They sent us to a birthing room where I managed to cope with my own contractions by deep breathing and meditation for about six hours. At that point, around 4 cm dilated, they said I was not making enough progress and they used the "p" word.

Pitocin is a synthetic form of oxytocin, a substance our bodies make that helps us progress through labor (and enjoy that after-sex glow). It is known, however, to cause severe contractions. I resisted for some time, but they kept insisting it was for the best. My water had broken, which meant Cub was in danger of the cord getting wrapped around his neck or an infection. Eventually, I relented and took the pit drip.

Within 20 minutes my contractions had become nearly unbearable, but I was determined to deliver as naturally as I could. I labored for six more hours with no pain relief as they continued to increase my Pitocin dosage. At around 9:35 a.m. I did something I never thought I would ever do... I begged for an epidural. The pain was so bad I could not breathe. Nothing I could do would ease it at all. Meanwhile, Jim was supporting me well, holding my hand, and talking with me quietly.

At 11 a.m. they had me coil up in a ball and they injected my lower back with pain medicine. The needle hurt so incredibly bad that I screamed. Jim just held me tighter, and we got through it. Less than 20 minutes later, I felt no pain, and I was able to talk and be my usual self for several hours, and it appeared that we were making some progress. Encouraged by cervical changes and Cub's positioning, I labored on and on.

Eventually, the epidural began wearing off. Within hours, it had very little impact on my pain. Although my legs were numb, dead weights, I still had horrific pain in my upper back. I progressed very slowly, getting all the way to 7 cm (with 10 cm needed for birth).

I stayed at 7 cm for five hours with no change. Then, during a cervical check, they found that Cub was facing up (just like my daughter). They made the decision to have a C-section. I burst into tears. A repeat C-section is the last thing I wanted! I was so happy when I found out I could try to VBAC. Vaginal births are better for Mom and baby. But worse, I had been laboring for 32 hours straight by this point. I feel like something was being taken from me.

At around 2 a.m. they wheeled me into the OR, which was only 25 steps from my room. The team was set up and ready to go. This was not an emergency, so we were able to go at a calm pace. As they pushed me from one table to another, I screamed in pain. My upper back was absolutely in utter agony. They couldn't give me medication to treat the pain, so after they placed me on the OR table, I did the only thing I could do: I asked Ganesh (remember that half-elephant guy I focus on during meditation?) to destroy the pain. Within 10 minutes, it was gone. It had been there for about 20 hours.

Soon Jim came in dressed in white scrubs. We were ready to bring our son into this world. As they began cutting, I heard them exclaim and mumble. It turns out that my uterus was absolutely covered in adhesions from the prior C-section. They had to take their time and be extremely careful as they cut through my uterus to take out my son. Then, I heard someone say, "It's a window." I know from my Mom's group that when the uterine scar stretches so thin you can see the baby inside the uterus, it's called a window.

Later, they would tell me they could clearly see Tristan's full head of hair through my uterine window! What that means is if I had made it to the pushing stage, we would have more than likely abrupted. If abruption had occurred, then Tristan and I both could have died...even at this incredible hospital. The scar tissues would have prevented a clean cut.

At some point during the cutting, they accidentally cut my bladder. It was full and stuck to my uterus. They repaired it after they

Tristan's (Cub's) Birth Story

delivered Cub. I am now wearing a Foley catheter around the clock for the next week. It will gently drain my bladder as it heals.

Meanwhile, I can feel them tugging and pulling on my uterus. At 2:55 a.m. on May 11, I hear the most wonderful sound in the world: Cub's big cry, quickly followed by, "Hey, he is peeing all over us!" (Cub really makes an entrance.) I could not see him. My face was covered by a sheet, but as they took him over to the incubator, Jim said he was stunning. As they sewed me back up, I anxiously awaited seeing his handsome face.

Just 10 minutes after he was born, the pediatrician announced that he scored a perfect 9/9 on Apgar score. Then, they placed him in Jim's arms. I cried when I saw his face. I have loved him so long. To be able to see him and know he is safe was overwhelming. Cub weighed 8 lbs. 15 oz. and was just beautiful. He had a bit of a glucose crash when he was born, but Daddy fed and burped him right beside me.

All went well for a while. I got to hold him for a while, and it was absolute bliss. He knew me right away, making eye contact for the ride over to our recovery room. I couldn't begin to describe what it felt like with him in my arms. He has a full head of hair and is stalky. We were a family for the first time!

Most of the wonder of the moment was lost when the pediatrician examining him found a blockage in his digestive tract. They were sending him to Children's Hospital. They were taking my baby away! I just got him in my arms!!! I began crying convulsively, hearing Jim explain to the team my history of child loss.

I was still unable to walk. At this point, I had been confined to a bed for 40+ hours. I was struggling with so much all at once. They wheeled me to my room and stopped by when it was time for them to take him the 20 minutes to Children's. He looked so good to me. I just couldn't believe he was sick.

Now, just two hours shy of the end of his first day of his life, I miss him more than any other person on Earth. I got to read him a story before he went to sleep, but I know he is longing for me as much as I am for him.

And that is how I became a mother.

About the author

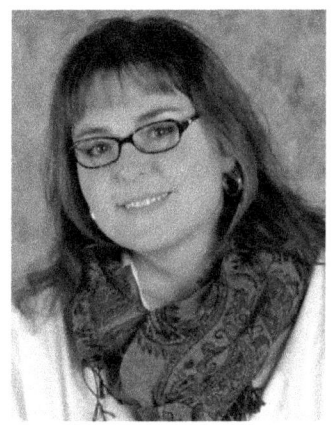

Photo by Karen Lyons.

DR. CHRISTINA (Fisanick) Greer is the author of more than 30 non-fiction books and multiple articles about writing. Two-Week Wait is her first book-length memoir. She has been teaching college writing for 20 years. Currently, she is an Associate Professor at California University of Pennsylvania, where she passes on her love of storytelling to future generations of writers and teachers. Christina lives in her home state of West Virginia with her two cats, husband, and son, who was worth every single two-week wait.

A note from the author

AS AN INDIE AUTHOR, I rely on readers like you to spread the word. If you could spare a few minutes to leave a review on Amazon, Goodreads, or wherever you talk about books with your friends, I would be eternally grateful.

www.ingramcontent.com/pod-product-compliance
Lightning Source LLC
LaVergne TN
LVHW041539070426
835507LV00011B/825